THE 7-DAY CARB CYCLE SOLUTION

CHOOSE TO LOSE:

THE 7-DAY CARB CYCLE SOLUTION

By Chris Powell

HYPERION

New York

A Stonesong Press Book

Copyright © 2012 by Chris Powell

All rights reserved. No part of this book may be used or reproduced in any manner whatsoever without the written permission of the Publisher. Printed in the United States of America. For information address Hyperion, 114 Fifth Avenue, New York, NY 10011.

Library of Congress Cataloging-in-Publication Data

Powell, Chris
 Choose to lose : the 7-day carb cycle solution / Chris Powell.
  p.cm
 1. Low-carbohydrate diet. I. Title.
 RM 237.73.P69 2011
 613.2'833—dc23
    2011025805

ISBN 978-1-4013-2445-2 (hardback)

Hyperion books are available for special promotions and premiums. For details contact the HarperCollins Special Markets Department in the New York office at 212-207-7528, fax 212-207-7222, or email spsales@harpercollins.com.

Designed by Mada Design, Inc. and produced by The Stonesong Press

FIRST EDITION

10 9 8 7 6 5 4 3

We try to produce the most beautiful books possible, and we are also extremely concerned about the impact of our manufacturing process on the forests of the world and the environment as a whole. Accordingly, we've made sure that all of the paper we use has been certified as coming from forests that are managed, to ensure the protection of the people and wildlife dependent upon them.

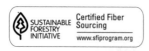

THIS LABEL APPLIES TO TEXT STOCK

DEDICATION

To my best friend and wife, Heidi: You are the love of my life, my soul mate, and my ultimate life coach. Your compassion for others has shown me a side of love that I didn't think existed. Every moment I get to spend with you is a gift. The hours, days, weeks, and years of collaboration on our vision to help others have been the most rewarding of my life. You are the hardest worker I have ever met. I wish the world could see the time, effort, insight, and sacrifice you have devoted to our vision. Simply put, without you, none of this would be a reality.

Heidi, I cashed in all of my karma chips for you. Thank you for loving me unconditionally and inspiring me daily to reach for the heavens. With you by my side, we will reach them.

ACKNOWLEDGMENTS

Thank you to my loving family, who gave me every opportunity in the world to learn and grow. Thank you for relentlessly encouraging me to follow my passion, even when I was too blind to see it. I get it now! Thank you to the amazing people who made this book possible: Gretchen Young, Elizabeth Sabo, Ellen Scordato, Constance Jones, Simon Green, and Ryan Levine. And a special thanks to my sister, whose articulate writing skills helped set the tone for this book.

Thank you to my teachers, professors, and coaches, who have opened my eyes to the beauty and durability of the human body. Thank you to my fellow trainers, who dedicate their lives to educating, motivating, and leading us to a life of health and happiness.

Thank you to the thousands of remarkable individuals who have trusted in me to guide you through your transformations. Thank you for believing. With your hope, dedication, and faith, you have made what once seemed impossible, possible. Thank you for allowing me to learn from your struggles and share in your victories. As you continue to change yourself, you are changing the lives of others around you. You create the momentum that keeps the message out there and continues to save more lives every day.

Thank you.

CONTENTS

It is advisable to consult a physician before starting any weight-loss plan. This program is not recommended for women who are pregnant or nursing.

PREFACE: MY STORY

The moment I started to grow into who I am today—a fitness expert and transformation coach—was the day I came home from school to find that my parents had taken the couches and chairs out of the living room and replaced them with a full weight-bench set. I was 14. The weight set was for me.

My family had just moved from Salinas, California, to Portland, Oregon, primarily because of my dad's job, but also because we could enjoy all kinds of outdoor activities there. Currently the oldest captain at Delta Airlines, my dad had been a navy fighter pilot and was really into physical fitness. My mom had always taken a holistic and organic approach to health and wellness. So clearing out their furniture and putting in a weight set was certainly new, but not an odd way to solve a family problem.

You see, I had always been the smallest kid in school. As a little kid, I was picked on by bullies. It's pretty easy to pick on the smallest kid. I realized that if I could get everyone in school to like me, my chances of being picked on were greatly reduced . . . so I compensated for my size with my personality. But that wasn't the problem.

The problem was that I wanted nothing more than to play football. A huge football fan, I used to go to San Francisco 49ers games with my grandpa. My old high school in Salinas didn't have a team, but my new school in Portland had one of the best in the state. Even though I was terrified by the prospect of being the new kid in school, I was thrilled that I was finally going to have an opportunity to play football.

Football practice started a week before classes and just two weeks after we'd moved to the area. I went out for football that week full of dreams and expectations—and quickly realized I was no match for the other kids. Drill after drill I found myself overpowered by the bigger, stronger guys. I dropped passes. I fumbled the ball every carry. I got laid out every rush. Players would push me aside at the drinking fountains and mock me in the huddle. It was devastating. On one hand, I loved having the chance to play. On the other hand, I was the smallest kid on the field by 40 or 50 pounds, and in no time flat the other kids let me know I was never going to be a part of their team. I quit after just one week.

My body was bruised, but my spirit was crushed.

Fortunately, I've been blessed to have parents whose philosophy is to provide opportunities, allow me to choose what I want to do, and encourage me to follow my passion. They saw how devastated I was after that week. Although I had always been small, for the first time ever I felt weak and powerless. They decided that the only way to turn this football disaster around was to help me to empower myself. Within a week, the weight set appeared in our living room.

For a week, I did nothing but sit on the bench press and watch the television, which was the only other thing left in the room. My daily pattern was to come home from school, drop my backpack on the floor, and sit down in front of the TV. When not watching TV, I spent the rest of my days moping around, uninspired to try anything new, especially working out. Even if I had been inspired, I really had no idea what to do with this huge contraption! It came with instructions, but at that point I wasn't interested in bridging the gap between seeing and doing.

One day, out of sheer boredom and a fleeting flash of curiosity, I sat down on the bench, lay down under the bar, and went through the motions of a bench press with just the bar, no weights. It felt heavy, but I did it. I wondered if I could do more by loading on some of the plates. I put weights on the bar, brought it down to my chest, and pushed it back up. I remember thinking, "I'm stronger than I thought I was!" For the first time since I'd been so destroyed on the football field, I felt good about myself because of what I could accomplish physically. I felt strong again.

That was the beginning. I realized that even though I was small, I could gain an edge if I was stronger and better developed. So I lifted, and lifted, and lifted. As the weeks went by, I was rapidly able to handle increasingly heavy weights. Seeing a tenfold increase in performance over the course of just a month made it easy for me to get hooked. I began to see a change in the size of my muscles as well and developed an identity among my peers as the smallest but strongest.

As much as I loved football, I became even more fascinated with how the human body can change. I became obsessed with pursuing my maximum potential. From my sophomore year on, I could always be found in the gym, either training myself or coaching someone else. I read all the bodybuilding magazines in a constant quest for bigger arms, a bigger chest, a higher vertical jump, a faster 40-yard dash.

After high school, I took my passion to Phoenix and enrolled at Arizona State University, which is ranked number two in the nation for what was then called exercise science and is now known as kinesiology. I took pre-med courses with a concentration on biomechanics and physiology, feeding my fascination with the awesome physiological mechanisms behind exercise science. But I didn't see a long-term career for myself in exercise science.

Since the age of 16, I had been taking flying lessons, and by 17 I had my private pilot's license. I subsequently got my instrument and commercial ratings and became a multi-engine flight instructor. I thought my best option for having a well-paying career was to follow my dad's footsteps into the world of commercial flying. Plus, I idolized my dad and thought it was the coolest thing in the world that he was a pilot.

I accrued over 1,200 hours flying time (which took almost seven years), but I was always uneasy flying. It never felt natural. I was always scared. It seemed like every time I flew, something went horribly wrong: electrical failures, engine problems, ruptured hydraulic lines, communications glitches, generator/alternator snafus, and the like. I got pretty good at handling emergencies, but I had to force myself to fly each and every day. A flying career just felt like the wrong path. Though my true path could not have been clearer, I continued to ignore it.

My first airline job interview was set for the morning of September 13, 2001—just two days after the tragic events of 9/11. Not surprisingly, the interview didn't happen. Instead, my life took a 180-degree turn. If the 9/11 terrorist attacks hadn't happened, I would likely be an airline pilot now. I would have remained on a path that wasn't for me. That awful event changed everything.

Within days, I got a job at a local gym and started as a personal trainer. It was like a thousand-pound weight had been lifted off my shoulders. I was alive! I was happy, doing what I love to do. Soon my skills were very much in demand, and I was fully booked as a trainer. I stopped flying altogether and began working on extra training certifications. Once I discovered the path I was meant to be on, my future unfolded in front of me. More and more opportunities appeared. It was awesome!

Within three short months, a business partner and I bought the personal training rights at a big gym next to Arizona State University. I hired a dream team of experienced and educated trainers, and for a couple of years we were the hottest training commodity in town. We trained everybody from arena football players, track athletes, bodybuilders, and cage fighters to stay-at-home moms and corporate executives.

Nothing beats raw, hands-on experience. I learned how to guide different kinds of people toward all kinds of fitness goals. This insight allowed me to create a multitude of fitness programs and apply my evolving principles to a wide range of challenges. Leading my clients to a better life was so rewarding. Their victories were like my own. Every client taught me valuable lessons in real-life health and fitness.

In early 2003, I became the resident fitness expert for *Good Morning Arizona* on Channel 3 in Phoenix. About five months later came another big turning point in my career. The producers received a letter from a viewer named David Smith, asking for my help. As I read his story, I became determined to help him. My work with David would become a very public weight-loss journey. I would soon be able to reveal to the world my unorthodox methods of personal transformation.

David was 26 years old and weighed 630 pounds. Just a year older than me, he was at risk of dying young. I had never worked with a morbidly obese client and wasn't sure what I was getting myself into. But I thought, "What if he just needs to know what to do?" After contacting him, I realized he had no money to pay me. Still, that didn't change my mind, and I started training him for free. I needed to make a living, but I could not live with the idea that David would continue to live in utter despair or even die. It became my mission to help him—simply because I could.

When I first met David, he was holed up in a basement. We immediately made a connection, and I could see that he sincerely wanted to make changes in his life. I saw him as an underdog, and I identified with that. We both had that "I'll show them" attitude.

With David's significant weight loss of 401 pounds in just under two years, I saw once again exactly how adaptable the human body is to nutrition and exercise, always adjusting to new conditions. If these two variables are manipulated in the right way, the result is consistent weight loss. I was just as excited to realize that weight loss did not have to stop, or plateau, before people reached their ideal weight. With this discovery and a renewed sense of purpose, I recommitted myself to helping as many people lose weight as I possibly could.

Since then, I've had the privilege of guiding hundreds of people through their weight-loss journeys. I've reached hundreds of thousands of people with *Extreme Makeover: Weight Loss Edition*, my television show on ABC. Every unique life transformation has taught me new and valuable lessons, not just about physical weight loss, but more importantly, about the power of the mind. When we look beyond the physical and discover our true potential within, weight loss can occur naturally. I have discovered the key to true and permanent transformation.

Now I want to share with you the secrets of discovering yourself and harnessing the power within you. I'll help you find your true identity, and I'll coach you step-by-step through the weight-loss journey—to a complete transformation of yourself!

CHAPTER ONE:
INTRODUCTION

According to government statistics, 70 percent of adults in the United States are overweight, including the 34 percent—a third of our population!—who are obese. Even more staggering is the rate of obesity among our children. No wonder more than half of all Americans have tried a weight-loss regimen at some point. Unfortunately, nine out of ten of us give up our weight-loss efforts within a week, often within the first three days. I witnessed this over and over again in my work as a personal trainer.

The National Institutes of Health (NIH) evaluates weight and overweight using a measure called Body Mass Index (BMI). BMI calculates the relationship between height and weight: The more you weigh relative to your height, the greater your BMI. Here's how it all adds up:

	Underweight (BMI under 18.5)	Healthy Weight (BMI 18.5–24.9)	Overweight (BMI 25–29.9)	Obese (BMI 30–39.9)	Morbidly Obese (BMI 40+)
Average Woman (5'4" tall)	under 110 lbs	110–144 lbs	145–173 lbs	174–232 lbs	over 232 lbs
Average Man (5'8" tall)	under 125 lbs	125–163 lbs	164–196 lbs	197–262 lbs	over 262 lbs

WEIGHING IN

What's your BMI? Visit www.nhlbisupport.com/bmi and use the BMI calculator or check the charts in Appendix A.

When I made nutrition plans for my clients, they'd at first think their program was fantastic. But three days or a week later, real life would set in, and they'd surrender. They couldn't hit their weight goals, so they ended up feeling like failures. For me, it felt as if I wasn't doing my job. I had failed to give my clients a plan they could stick with. How to break through that three-day to one-week failure wall? I was determined to find the secret to sustainable weight loss and the keys to improving physical health and emotional well-being. I had to make weight loss easy, fast, and fun.

I knew it was possible to stay motivated for more than a few days or a week, but I also knew we each have a unique, individual, and super-busy life. It became clear to me that all too often our habitual lifestyle doesn't facilitate weight loss. To lose weight permanently, I realized, we must embrace a new lifestyle. To embrace a new lifestyle, we must be equipped with the right mindset, the right knowledge, and the right tools.

A light bulb went off in my head. I realized what my clients needed to know and what tools they needed to make sustainable change in their lives. I started to design a whole new way to lose weight. Now, after years of hard work and incredible results with my clients, I've created a program—The Carb-Cycle Solution—that's effective for everyone.

YOU CAN LOSE WEIGHT

If you work it, The Carb-Cycle Solution will work for you, for the rest of your life. As you change your lifestyle, you'll quickly realize that you *can* lose weight and keep it off. You'll see the results you want and quite possibly surpass your expectations.

My program, The Carb-Cycle Solution, is a unique twist on the powerful weight-loss method called carb cycling. Essentially, it's a system for eating a high-carbohydrate diet one day followed by a low-carbohydrate diet the next. Alternating high-carb days with low-carb days is a wonderfully balanced nutrition technique. It's easy to follow because you don't feel deprived, and it can bring you amazing and permanent weight-loss results.

There is a reason why I work with the super obese: They have a longer journey than any of us, but they are able to completely transform their bodies and change their lives within just one or two short years. They are living proof of the body and mind's amazing ability to transform. And if they can do it, anyone can do it: especially you.

THE SCARIEST FOUR-LETTER WORD: DIET

Ah, the word "diet." It probably makes you think of restriction, deprivation, and boredom, among other disagreeable things. I want you to rethink this four-letter word. The word *diet* simply refers to a pattern of eating. That's it! You can have a 5,000-calorie-a-day diet, or a 1,500-calorie-a-day diet. Some diets are high in protein and low in carbohydrates, and some diets are high in carbohydrates and low in fats. There are diets that are high in pizza and low in vegetables. The way you eat right now is your diet.

You're reading this book, so chances are that your current diet—your pattern of eating—isn't working for you. You've taken the first step toward *choosing* to make changes to your diet. Awesome! As the old saying goes, "If you always do what you've always done, then you'll always get what you've always got." It's so brilliantly simple and true, especially when it comes to the way you eat.

The many popular diets out there have similar themes. They're about counting calories, limiting carbohydrates or fats or meats, following the glycemic index, watching portion sizes, eating in specific ratios, and on and on. Please don't get me wrong: These programs include some bright ideas. They're popular because in one form or another, they've proven successful for some people. But it can be easier!

WHAT'S THE DIFFERENCE?

I have designed The Carb-Cycle Solution with long-term practicality in mind. I don't want you to lose weight for just a year; I want you to lose weight for a lifetime. Along with hundreds of my clients, I have been following this plan for many years with ease.

The Carb-Cycle Solution takes the best from the most effective diets out there and puts a real-life twist on the concepts. Real people with real lives and real weight to lose can easily follow my plan. It not only stimulates weight loss, it works emotionally and psychologically, banishing feelings of deprivation and limitation. You'll eat whole, healthy foods and reward yourself with cheat foods as often as every other day. And you don't have to count calories or figure out the glycemic index. This no-nonsense practical approach simplifies nutrition to make it fast, easy, and fun.

The key to The Carb-Cycle Solution, and what most distinguishes it from traditional diets, is its colossal improvement over the others: It doesn't let your body adapt to a monotonous diet and exercise routine. Yet it's so incredibly easy to do. You simply alternate between high-carb days and low-carb days. This tricks your body into maximizing fat loss, conquering the dieter's plateau, and bringing long-term weight loss. You'll drop pounds safely and quickly and learn how to optimize your overall health and fitness.

Another plus of The Carb-Cycle Solution is that you can fine-tune it to suit your needs. You can reach your goal in a couple ways: over a long period of time with lots of flexibility, or in a shorter, more rigorous interval. Either way, the program empowers you to create the body you've always wanted . . . while you eat the foods you enjoy! You'll be astounded at how easy it can be to keep your new, fantastic physique for the rest of your life. You are in control.

YOUR LIFE CYCLE

The Carb-Cycle Solution consists of only two parts. The 7-Day Carb Cycle (see Chapter 9) boosts your metabolism so your body can burn fat rapidly. You simply alternate days when you eat a high-carbohydrate diet with days when you eat a low-carbohydrate diet. If you ever hit the dieter's plateau and your weight loss slows or stops, the Slingshot Technique (see Chapter 11) changes up the carb cycling pattern to re-start your metabolism, so you can lose even more. In both stages, you have complete control over your nutrition, plus plenty of opportunities to indulge.

It's no secret that the most phenomenal weight-loss success stories start with not only good nutrition but also exercise. Along with carb cycling, you'll start a workout program that you can easily fit into your lifestyle, preferably first thing in the morning for best results. For strength training and body-shaping, on your low-carb days you'll do basic exercises that I call *shapers*. Each shaper workout takes only 10 minutes, and you can do it almost anywhere. Six days a week you'll do cardiovascular workouts that I call *shredders*. These are intervals of low-, moderate-, and high-intensity cardio exercise that take just 6 minutes each. Shredders optimize fat burning.

The Carb-Cycle Solution nutrition and exercise program works in 90-day phases. Each month in a phase consists of three 7-Day Carb Cycles plus one Slingshot week, and from one month to the next you increase the intensity of your workouts.

You should notice a difference in the way you look and feel less than a week after you start The Carb-Cycle Solution. How long it takes to reach your goal weight depends on how much weight you want to lose. If you're looking to drop 30 pounds, you can probably reach your goal with one 90-day phase. If you need to lose 150 pounds, it may take several phases to get there in a healthy way.

LET'S GO!

Along with the nuts and bolts of The Carb-Cycle Solution program, this book contains a wealth of insider tips and tricks to keep you motivated, plus ways to chart your progress. Transformation is as much about the mind as it is about the body. Choosing to make a change is the first and most important part of The Carb-Cycle Solution. By picking up this book, you're already heading in the right direction.

You're at the beginning of an exhilarating journey, and I'll be by your side to help you become who you *really* are. Along the way, we'll celebrate your victories, big and small. So let's get started—it's going to be fast, easy, and fun.

My heartfelt welcome to you!

CHAPTER 2:
DAVID'S STORY

One fateful day in June 2003, I received an email that would change my life forever.

"My name is David Smith. I have an all too common name but I am not at all common . . . I am 26 years old and I weigh over 630 pounds. I gained most of my weight drinking soda. I used to drink more than four liters a day of it. My favorite foods are ice cream, pizza and pizza again. I have tried lots of diets, but they have never worked. . . .

"I started to gain weight when I was 5 years old. Nobody knew at the time that I, a chubby 5-year-old, would turn into a morbidly obese man. But I did. I was never good at making friends. I have only had a few in my life and I have never had a girlfriend, mostly because I was ashamed of myself. I was very shy. . . .The first friend I ever had was abusive toward me. . . . I was molested by a friend, my only friend. I have been picked on all my life. I turned to food and soda at an early age because it doesn't judge me, it doesn't hurt me and it made me feel good.

"Halfway through 11th grade I was 17 years old and 375 pounds. I couldn't handle being around people anymore and I dropped out of school. . . . Almost 10 years of my life was wasted since then and I have done nothing at all. I don't have a single friend. I was afraid of the outside world, so I would stay in my house (my prison) day and night. I was afraid to go into my back yard until it was dark out. . . .

"Seven years ago my mother was diagnosed with Non-Hodgkin's Lymphoma. . . . My family and I took care of her the best we could at the end, but I almost needed help too because of my weight. She died almost two years ago and it hit me hard. The first month I hardly ate anything, but after the first month I was an eating machine. I didn't care about anything. I just wanted to get my fix and be left alone. . . .

"I was even planning on ending my life. I was weeks from doing it when my father told me that the reason he keeps going is because of me. That shot through me like a lightning bolt. I didn't realize that he loved me and that if I did take my life it would devastate him. I was at the crossroads of my life and I chose the right road. . . . I abandoned my suicide plans for good.

"I have haunted my house like a ghost for 10 years and I don't want to haunt it anymore. I decided to put it all behind me and start my life over. I think I might be able to inspire others to do the same. It makes me feel good just thinking about it. There are a lot of things I have never experienced in my life, and there are a lot of opportunities I want to explore. The life I have been living is false. It is not for me anymore. My destiny is something else.

"Please call or email me soon. Thank you.

David E. Smith Jr."

DETERMINATION

After reading David's message, I knew I could help him. In fact, I knew that I had to help this man.

The first day I showed up to train David, I was taken aback by his massive size. When he opened the door, it occurred to me that he was about the size of a small car. I had only seen or heard of people that large on television. His legs were like massive tree trunks, and he was so wide he could barely fit through a doorway. I couldn't imagine how he functioned with such an enormous body, and soon I learned that he really *didn't* function. For him, life was about getting from morning to night without hurting himself out of deep shame and sorrow. As if his enormous body was not enough, David suffered from other physical difficulties. He wore very thick glasses due to extreme near-sightedness, and he had an obvious overbite. An entire mouthful of yellow teeth in bad condition was the result of eating and drinking all the wrong foods for many years.

As I looked at David for the first time, I couldn't help but wonder if he had the dedication it would take to reverse his condition. But after speaking with him for only 15 minutes, I *knew* that I could help him. He didn't have an eating problem. He had a timing problem—he ate at the wrong times. David went all day without eating (just drinking soda), and then he gorged himself at night. He wanted to change; he just didn't know how to do it or where to start. I knew he could lose the weight fast. He simply needed the path laid out for him.

In David's case, there was a psychological and emotional need for food late at night. I knew I needed to approach his weight loss delicately and still allow him to eat the foods that he felt comfortable with. Most importantly, I knew he was determined to make a change in his life. His resolve to start fresh by regaining his health reignited my belief in the human spirit.

REVVING UP

The beauty of David's situation was that because of his size, he was in a position to maximize his metabolic potential and drop weight rapidly. It seems counterintuitive, but the heavier you are, the higher your metabolic potential. Many of my overweight clients come to me with the misconception that they're overweight because of a sluggish metabolism. It's as if they're sitting on a V8 engine, but they don't know how to rev it up! With David, I was dealing with a V12.

Making David's nutrition plan, I simply restructured the way he ate and gave him easy guidelines to follow. He was still allowed to eat his favorite foods, but we kept it on a schedule at specific reward times. I introduced real food—lean proteins, complex carbohydrates, and green vegetables—into his diet. David also began eating five meals every day instead of just one or two.

As part of his weight-loss protocol, David began carbohydrate cycling. The system was easy for him, because if he wanted or craved a certain food, he could either time his meals to eat it today, or he could always choose to have it tomorrow. Within a month of starting my program, he dropped more than 30 pounds.

We began working out soon after he had mastered the nutrition program. At first, it was everything David could do to get out of a chair. It took him about 30 seconds to stand up from a sitting position. So his initial workouts were getting up and down from the couch and walking one lap around his small block. He needed to learn how to move in everyday life. He needed to become functional again. When we first started walking, I had to watch his footing carefully because he literally could not see the ground in front of him. He could have easily stepped off a curb and broken his foot. Our short walks required focus from me and hard work from him.

As David built up his stamina, I added stair climbing to his regimen. He would walk up his stairs and guide himself back down with the rail. At first, he'd have to sit down at the top and rest for a while after walking up his stairs. But with each session he became stronger, and he was eventually able to turn right around and come back down, then go up again. To finish our sessions, I had David lie on the floor and guided him through some core exercises—movements that would strengthen his abdomen and lower back muscles.

BREAKING THROUGH THE PLATEAU

After a few months of eating the right foods in the right way and working out at his own pace, David saw his weight loss slow down. He had lost almost 150 pounds but could not break through the 480-pound mark. We were stuck there for three or four weeks. At first, I reduced David's calorie intake slightly and increased his exercise intensity to see how his body would react. Nothing.

I finally sat down with David and asked exactly what he had been eating. As we analyzed his nutrition regimen, I realized he had slipped back into thinking that to lose weight faster, he needed to keep eating less. At 480 pounds, he had slowly reduced his calorie intake and carbs to such low levels that his metabolism had slowed down and his body had halted his weight loss. He was exercising so much every day that his body was overstressed.

I took a deep breath and said, "David . . . bear with me here: I'm going to ask you to do something that will seem completely out of the ordinary—but you have to follow my advice. Get a good video game and conquer it for the next two weeks, because you and I are not going to work out. Instead, double the amount you're eating every day." He looked at me like I had gone completely insane. Then he shrugged and said, "Okay, if you're sure."

"I'll call you in two weeks," I said, and I left.

In those two weeks, David dropped more than 20 pounds. I knew I had hit upon something huge. His weight loss had plateaued because his body had adapted to the nutrition and exercise program. To break through that barrier his body needed to relax, reset, and release. Over two weeks, his body had retuned and re-boosted his metabolism. He started cycling his carbohydrates again after two weeks, and he was right back on track, dropping about 30 pounds each month. Every time his weight loss stalled, we would simply take a week to reset him and get him right back on track . . . all the way to his goal weight.

SHARING THE VICTORY

After two years and 401 pounds lost, David became the man he wanted to be . . . and that I had believed he could be. He also became an inspirational media star. You might have seen him on *Oprah, 20/20,* or *The View.* More important to me, he became one of my best friends.

Almost a year and a half after I started helping David, he handed me a note following one of our sessions.

"I am writing this today at 330 pounds, a 300-pound difference from my starting weight. My life, my world and my existence have changed dramatically since I first met you. You showed me the way to my freedom, and I am glad you did because if you didn't, I probably wouldn't be here.

"I never thought losing weight would be this easy. I am losing weight quicker than someone with a gastric bypass. The only thing I needed was commitment. At first I couldn't walk 500 feet without stopping. Now I can walk miles without stopping.

"I have recently started to regain a life that I never thought I could have. I am no longer that scared little boy; I am starting to become the confident man I knew I could be. I have finally obtained my driver's license. Seven months ago I couldn't even fit in the front seat of a car. I am working on getting my GED and I also want to look for my first job.

"I am not afraid of people anymore. Even though I'm still a big guy, I can walk with my head held high. I finally love myself. If you love yourself you can be anything you want to be. I can't wait to experience the things that I have never experienced in my life. I want to experience a lot of things that are fun, adventurous, exciting, mysterious and dangerous. I have only allowed myself to experience pain and suffering. The one thing that I am most excited about experiencing is love. I have heard that the greatest feeling in life is to fall in love. I want to know how that feels.

"No matter how deep you dig yourself into a hole, you can always dig yourself out. I am proof of that. Nothing is impossible in this world. If you want it you just need to grab hold of it and never let go . . . because some dreams really do come true."

I read David's note in the middle of a coffee shop and cried for half an hour. I had to show off his victory. The news channel on which I regularly appeared heard about my work with David and asked to follow his progress on the air. So with a little hesitation and a lot of courage, he agreed to share his struggles and triumphs with hundreds of thousands of people. Since then, his remarkable 401-pound, 22-month weight loss has drawn millions of eyes to TLC's television documentary, *The Six-Hundred-Fifty-Pound Virgin*, which first aired in May 2009. David's story continues to inspire millions.

I admire David's desire to show people how he lived at nearly 650 pounds and what motivated him to transform. He wants nothing more than to encourage others to use his story as an example, and eventually, to celebrate their own incredible accomplishments. David's courage has sparked a tremendous movement; he's accomplishing his noble goal.

PART ONE:
DISCOVERY

CHAPTER 3:
WHY AM I OVERWEIGHT?

You're a human being. Thanks to advances in the field of genetics, we've learned an incredible amount about what that means. Analysis of the DNA from a single strand of your hair can tell you a great deal about your body and where you came from. Pretty amazing stuff!

FROM FORAGING TO FARMING

One thing we humans have in common is that our prehistoric ancestors were survivors. They fought predators, enemies, disease, famines, and sometimes extreme climates. They endured harsh conditions generation after generation after generation. If early humans weren't able to overcome the challenges they faced, their bloodline died out. Only those who could adapt to difficult, changing circumstances lived long enough to procreate.

At the beginning of human existence, our prehistoric ancestors lived off the land, foraging for plants and hunting animals to ensure their survival. Their bodies had to be lean and strong in order to obtain the food they needed, and in fact, the way they ate and lived helped keep them that way. Weather, animal migration, and other forces of nature made it hard to know when food would be available. Our prehistoric ancestors' bodies learned to adjust to these variables, conserving fat and reducing the calories they used to survive during famines. Those primitive bodies were brilliant!

People did less hunting and gathering when they began growing and harvesting crops and raising domesticated animals. This shift, which occurred over thousands of years, meant that food was easier to come by. Nevertheless, the farming lifestyle was extremely rigorous. To produce food to feed the family, you gotta work the farm all day! Physical fitness was the natural result of both daily survival and a diet of fresh food grown by the people who ate it.

As humans and their tools, clothing, and shelter evolved, they also had to adapt to new foods. Digestive adaptation? Absolutely.

INDUSTRIALIZED EATING

Most Americans had a farming lifestyle all the way up to the start of the Industrial Revolution about 200 years ago. The new era was a time of major change in human history. As people left farms and villages and moved to cities to work in factories, society transitioned from predominantly rural to predominantly urban. Steam and electric power, the automobile, and the factory assembly line all began to reduce the amount of physical labor we needed to survive. At the same time, there was a huge increase in the population.

The next big population explosion occurred after World War II when soldiers returned home and started families. The food industry had more people to feed, and food became a big business. In order to meet the increased demand for food, they began producing processed "convenience" food to feed the masses.

And so the human digestive system was introduced to "fast" processed foods. I call them fast foods because processing removes much of food's fiber and nutrients, allowing it to be digested quickly. The digestive system once took hours to break down food and send nutrients into the bloodstream; now it took just minutes. Fast foods put people at risk for serious health problems: They released dangerously high levels of sugars and fats into the blood, which wreaked havoc on the body's organs.

What's more, to enhance flavor the food industry began adding sodium, sugar, and fats to this partially pre-digested processed food. The move increased sales but also increased waistlines . . . and food addiction. Never before in history had our bodies experienced such an overload of sugar, fat, and sodium. Food became the feel-good fix for many, leading to emotional, psychological, and even physical dependence upon processed foods.

Things only got worse in the late 1970s and early 1980s. The United States government stepped up farm subsidies, increasing supplies of corn, wheat, and soybeans. Since these crops are largely used in the manufacture of processed foods, the cost of processed foods went down. But the government didn't subsidize the farming of fruits and vegetables, so the cost of healthy, fresh produce went up by 40 percent in the same period! Not good. Basically, junk food got cheap, and healthy food expensive.

For the first time in history, the amount of food we produced and the availability of that food far exceeded our needs. We could get whatever we wanted to eat, and our daily calorie intake started to rise dramatically. At the same time, marketing of all this processed food escalated. According to government statistics, $31 billion is spent every year to advertise fast foods and processed foods, as opposed to $2 billion spent on marketing natural foods like fresh fruits and vegetables, dairy products, and quality meat. Many processed foods are being marketed with catchy slogans about health benefits, or they're touted as preventing weight-related illnesses. We're being manipulated to *think* we're eating well when actually, we're not.

FAST AND FAT

Unfortunately, processed foods have become the norm in our diets—just look around your supermarket. It's horrifying to see the next generation growing up on fast foods, not knowing or understanding the benefits of real, whole food. Just a single soda or large latte brims with 200 empty calories. The typical fast-food cheeseburger packs 300 calories. Day after day, year after year, all these calories turn into a weight gain of 50 pounds . . . 100 pounds . . . or more!

Healthy food has become a mystery to many Americans. I meet a lot of people who ask me, "Don't you ever eat *normal* food?" It surprises me, because I realize they're referring to fast food and processed food as normal. This distorted viewpoint reveals the power of marketing and the muscle of the gigantic food industry. It's not about health anymore; it's all about the money. Since when did whole, natural foods become abnormal?! We've forgotten where we come from: As humans, we require real, whole, natural foods to sustain our health. So I answer the question by declaring, "Yes, I do eat normal human food!"

Most recently, we've left the Industrial Age behind and have entered the Information Age. Computer work has mostly replaced physical factory labor, and our jobs have become increasingly sedentary. Technology hasn't just reduced activity in the workplace. It has taken over our homes. Most of us now spend the majority of our days sitting in front of a screen of some kind or another.

On the face of it, machines and computers have made our lives easier. New devices and increasingly sophisticated software make it possible for us to do more work in less time. So what do we do with all that extra time? Fill it with more work. C'mon, this is America; we built this country on hard work! Productivity in the workplace is all-important.

Hard work is commendable, but it's a problem when we're connected 24/7. We've become a people who never stop to watch the sunset, to enjoy the beauty of the world around us, or to focus on our own health and happiness. We are too busy multi-tasking with our smartphones and laptops. We eat fast foods on the run or starve ourselves before bolting down huge meals. Our over-scheduled and stressed-out lifestyles have ruined our health.

HOW TO GROW A HUMAN

Until the 20th century, modifications to our diet happened very, very gradually. But in the last couple of generations, we've changed our eating habits at an ever-accelerating rate. Our great-grandparents could not have imagined microwave brownies or drive-through burritos. What we eat has changed more in the last 50 years than in the previous 5,000 years. It's staggering!

Even with our incredible ability to adapt, there's no way our bodies can keep up with such rapid change. It takes hundreds of generations for our DNA to change by less than 0.01 percent, and it would take about 500 generations for our bodies to adapt to the dietary changes that have taken place in just the last two generations. This is why, for the first time in human existence, we're faced with a monumental obesity pandemic.

Americans now eat like Japanese sumo wrestlers. Yes, I *did* just say sumo wrestlers. Let me explain.

Ever see a sumo wrestler before he begins initial training? He's a 150-pound beanpole! But within several years, sumo wrestlers become 400-pound behemoths. Many young men enter sumo training-stables as scrawny little runts, hoping to end up as quarter-ton wrestling gods. To gain all that glorious weight, they must follow a strict regimen: They get up early and train hard for several hours on an empty stomach. They starve until the afternoon, when they eat an enormous 3,000 to 4,000 calorie meal of meat, fish, vegetables, lard, and rice, often washed down with beer. Then they take a nap. In the evening, they have another similar meal of even more calories (5,000–6,000) before going to bed.

Unconsciously, we've adopted similar eating habits. We get up with the alarm clock and rush out to work on an empty stomach, grabbing a huge cup of coffee from the local java joint on the way. After slaving away all morning, in early afternoon we realize we're starving and go out to shovel down a high-calorie lunch. Unlike the sumo wrestlers, who can nap, we have to push through the mid-afternoon slump. So when we leave work we're exhausted and hungry again. We stop at the drive-through or order in pizza, then sit in front of the TV, often snacking, until we fall asleep. Sounds familiar, doesn't it?

It's the perfect recipe for growing a human. This is why it happens.

Number one, we don't eat breakfast, which stresses our bodies and releases high levels of cortisol. What does cortisol do? It stimulates our bodies to gain belly fat. On top of this massive cortisol surge, we release even *more* cortisol by loading up on caffeine all day, stressing our bodies to the max. This ensures that our next meal will end up as soft, squishy fat in the last place we want it.

Number two, skipping breakfast and eating only two big meals a day slows the metabolism to a crawl. Research has shown that this triggers stronger cravings and increases the likelihood of overeating later in the day.

The last ingredient in the weight-gain recipe is going to sleep right after eating huge meals. When we sleep, our metabolism slows, so eating lots of calories before bedtime enables our bodies to store them as fat rather than use them as energy.

This trifecta of bad habits—skipping breakfast, eating two big meals a day, and stuffing ourselves late in the day—works like a charm to grow a human being to the larger and larger sizes that a sumo wrestler works for years to attain. Without thinking, we're becoming a nation of sumo wrestlers. None of us wants to be fat, but it seems we do everything we can to gain weight. Our typical everyday lifestyle is, accidentally, one of the fastest methods for weight gain.

CHAPTER 4:
THE FURNACE

Although the scientific study of weight loss is still getting underway, there's a lot that we already *do* know about how the human body uses calories. To understand weight gain and weight loss, we need to look at the physics of our physique. Consider the First Law of Thermodynamics, which states that energy cannot be created or destroyed; it can only be transferred. Every body obeys this basic law of physics—no exceptions.

To make it simple, think of your body as a furnace. It burns the energy (calories) from food, just as a furnace burns the energy from fuel. Your body converts—transfers—calories into cellular function, heat, and movement. A furnace converts fuel into heat. If your body takes in more calories than it needs to function, it stores the excess by transferring it into fat.

At the most basic level, to maintain your weight you must consume the same number of calories as your metabolic furnace burns. To gain weight you must consume more calories, and to lose weight you must consume fewer calories. Simple, right? Keep reading. You're gonna learn some cool stuff!

ENERGY TO BURN

To start off, let's take a look at approximately how many calories you use in a day. Your body uses calories even when it's at rest. The baseline measurement of your daily caloric requirement is called Resting Metabolic Rate (RMR). This is a calculation of how many calories your body would burn if you lay perfectly still for 24 hours.

The moment you begin to move in the morning, your muscles begin burning calories to function. Your abdominal muscles contract to sit up in bed, and your leg muscles contract as you place your feet on the floor and stand up to walk to the bathroom. This symphony of muscular movement continues throughout the day, burning more calories every time you move your muscles. In addition, digesting your food alone burns one to three hundred more calories every day.

These two charts, for men and women, give an estimate of how many calories your body burns every day with little to no activity. Find your number and circle it.

CALORIES BURNED DAILY: **AVERAGE MAN** AT 5'8" TALL	WEIGHT	20 years	30 years	40 years	50 years	60 years	70 years	80 years
	125 – 150	2318.483	2230.408	2142.333	2054.258	1966.183	1878.108	1790.033
	150 – 175	2521.608	2433.533	2345.458	2257.383	2169.308	2081.233	1993.158
	175 – 200	2724.733	2636.658	2548.583	2460.508	2372.433	2284.358	2196.283
	200 – 250	3130.983	3042.908	2954.833	2866.758	2778.683	2690.608	2602.533
	250 – 300	3334.108	3246.033	3157.958	3069.883	2981.808	2893.733	2805.658
	300 – 350	3740.358	3652.283	3564.208	3476.133	3388.058	3299.983	3211.908
	350 – 400	4146.608	4058.533	3970.458	3882.383	3794.308	3706.233	3618.158
	400 – 500	4755.983	4667.908	4579.833	4491.758	4403.683	4315.608	4227.533

CALORIES BURNED DAILY: **AVERAGE WOMAN** AT 5'4" TALL	WEIGHT	20 years	30 years	40 years	50 years	60 years	70 years	80 years
	100 – 125	1827.369	1766.581	1705.793	1645.005	1584.217	1523.429	1462.641
	125 – 150	1968.64	1907.852	1847.064	1786.276	1725.488	1664.7	1603.912
	150 – 175	2109.912	2049.124	1988.336	1927.548	1866.76	1805.972	1745.184
	175 – 200	2251.184	2190.396	2129.608	2068.82	2008.032	1947.244	1886.456
	200 – 250	2533.727	2472.939	2412.151	2351.363	2290.575	2229.787	2168.999
	250 – 300	2674.998	2614.21	2553.422	2492.634	2431.846	2371.058	2310.27
	300 – 350	2957.541	2896.753	2835.965	2775.177	2714.389	2653.601	2592.813
	350 – 400	3240.085	3179.297	3118.509	3057.721	2996.933	2936.145	2875.357
	400 – 500	3663.899	3603.111	3542.323	3481.535	3420.747	3359.959	3299.171

For example, I'm 33 years old and weigh 185 pounds. The chart shows that on an average day, with very light activity, my body furnace would burn about 2,636 calories in 24 hours. To lose weight, I would need to consume less than 2,636 calories. To gain weight, I would need to consume more than that. Get it? Good!

Now, let's say I want to lose one pound of fat, which equals 3,500 calories. How long will it take? If I choose to eat 2,136 calories daily, my body would still need 2,636 calories to function, so it would be 500 calories short and would burn 500 calories from its own living tissue . . . body fat. In seven days, it would burn 3,500 calories, or one pound, of fat. If I choose to eat even less, my daily calorie deficit would be bigger, and I would lose body fat faster. Get it? Good!

HOW WEIGHT IS LOST

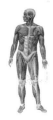 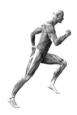 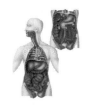

| Resting Metabolic Rate | Physical Activity | Feeding & Digestion |
| 60-75% of daily calories burned | 20-35% of daily calories burned | 10-15% of daily calories burned |

2,636 calories burned daily

500 extra calories burned

2,136 calories consumed daily

Protein, Carbohydrates, and Fats

1 Pound of Body Fat = 3,500 Calories

7 Days Burning 500 Extra Calories = 1 Pound Lost

THE METABOLIC MIRACLE

So why is it that some people can eat absolutely anything and never gain a pound? They may eat upwards of 2,500 to 3,500 calories a day, and they're still lean and slender. Meanwhile, folks on the other side of the spectrum struggle to lose weight, yet eat only 1,200 to 1,500 calories a day. Doesn't seem fair, does it? Well, I can explain. The secret behind this paradox is that your metabolism always adjusts to your food intake.

Let me pose some questions to you: Have you tried to lose weight before, only to end up frustrated when it didn't work or when the weight came back on? Have you tried and failed to overcome your slowed or stalled weight loss with diets? Do you skip meals? Do you currently eat a very low-calorie diet? Have you eliminated carbohydrates? If you answered "yes" to any of these questions, you need to open your eyes to how your metabolism uses energy and how you can convince your body to lose weight.

The way your body burns energy is roughly referred to as your *metabolism*. Metabolism, the metabolic furnace, is a broad term that refers to all the life-sustaining chemical reactions in your body. It's usually measured in terms of calories. The Greek word *metabol*, the root of metabolism, literally means "change." Your metabolism changes according to the conditions you impose upon it. Eat less and your metabolic furnace cools down. Eat more and it heats up. You can manipulate your metabolism to accelerate weight loss. You can stoke your metabolic furnace to burn MUCH hotter, so it burns way more calories than the baseline shown in the charts. The hotter it gets, the more fuel it burns. The more fuel it burns, the faster your body shrinks!

So the million-dollar question is, HOW DO YOU MAKE YOUR FURNACE BURN THE HOTTEST SO YOU CAN LOSE FAT THE FASTEST?

I've got the solution.

RULE 1: Eat more often.

RULE 2: Eat carbohydrates.

RULE 3: Build muscle.

RULE 4: Move your muscles.

Losing weight can be more difficult (but not impossible) if you're predisposed to hormone imbalances or if you're at a stage of life when hormonal effects are changing. If either of these is the case, it's advisable to get a medical diagnosis and seek help to balance your hormones so you can safely reach your weight-loss goals. But as much as we would like to blame our weight issues on our hormones, the raw truth is that for most of us, our lifestyle is actually what needs balancing!

EAT MORE OFTEN

The best way to kindle your body's metabolic furnace from smoldering ash to a blazing inferno is to eat a perfectly portioned meal every 3 hours. These smaller, more frequent meals step up the heat to incinerating levels.

If you follow The Carb-Cycle Solution, you restart your furnace every morning. Breakfast lights the fire. Three hours later, you feed it more fuel. And again. And again. And again. Soon your furnace is burning so hot that even if you eat a huge meal, essentially throwing a large shot of fuel into the furnace, it will quickly burn up.

What happens if you stop feeding the furnace? It cools down. Well, what happens when you feed a furnace lots of fuel after it has cooled down? The fuel doesn't burn; it just sits there. If you allow too much time to go by without eating, your body will cool down its metabolism to conserve energy. It'll hang onto extra fuel in the form of fat. Remember the sumo wrestlers? This is how they trick their metabolism so they can gain maximum weight! If they started eating every three hours, they'd stoke their metabolic furnace to a raging firestorm and lose fat quickly!

Your body will always adapt to match metabolic burn with food intake. Eat 2,500–3,000 calories throughout the day, and your body will attempt to stoke its metabolic furnace to incinerate that many calories. Eat 1,200 or fewer calories throughout the day, and over time, your metabolism will drop to match. This is why you see immediate and often significant weight gain if you fall off the wagon of typical weight-loss programs. Your metabolism is as low as possible when you're in a starvation state, so when you eat a lot of calories it can't burn them, resulting in weight gain. When you see this happening, your knee-jerk reaction might be to starve again to get back on track, but this further cools down your metabolism . . . and the yo-yo dieting disaster begins.

There's another reason to feed your furnace often. Believe it or not, the simple act of eating stimulates your metabolism by triggering digestion! Every time your body digests food, it ramps up your total metabolic rate.

Scientists call this *food-induced thermogenesis*. (In Greek, "thermo" means "heat" and "genesis" means "make.") The process accounts for about 10 percent of the calories your body burns daily. From the moment you swallow that first bite of food at breakfast, your digestive system demands a share of the heat generated by your metabolism.

EAT CARBOHYDRATES

Each of the main macronutrients—proteins, carbohydrates, and fats—helps your body to maximize its function. Proteins are the building blocks for nearly all the tissues in your body and actually require the most energy to digest. Fats help regulate hormone balance, assist with hair and nail growth, and promote healthy cellular function. But carbohydrates . . . that's where the magic happens. They're not only the primary fuel for your cells, but they also indirectly affect your body's metabolic thermostat.

Your thyroid is the thermostat on your metabolic furnace. It releases hormones that play a major role in controlling your body temperature and the rate at which your body burns calories. When your thyroid's working at its max, your metabolic rate is sky-high, and you're a fat-burning furnace. If thyroid function is impaired, your metabolic rate slows. This can happen when you don't eat enough carbohydrates. Add carbs back into your diet, and your metabolic thermostat cranks back up. Carbs keep your metabolic thermostat set to high!

METABOLIC MUSCLE

The good news about your metabolism is that your body uses energy on a grand scale even when you're resting. From your resting muscles to your beating heart to your breathing lungs, your body is burning calories all the time. This adds up to 60–75 percent of the calories you burn in a day!

Every moment of every day, your organs steadily consume energy. But the single largest consumer of calories in your body is . . . drum roll . . . YOUR MUSCLE! You have billions of muscle cells, the most active living tissue in your body. The more muscle you have, the hotter your body's furnace burns, even when you're asleep. This is why it's imperative to focus on maintaining and building muscle during your weight-loss transformation. More muscle will get you to your goal in a fraction of the time!

How do we maintain or gain muscle? We do resistance training (often called weight training or strength training), which stimulates our muscles to grow and define their shapes. The Carb-Cycle Solution includes a fast and fun 10-minute body weight resistance Shaper every other morning. These exercises help stoke your metabolic furnace to accelerate weight loss.

MUSCLE IN MOTION

Your muscles require a ton of calories to sustain them at rest, and as soon as you start moving them, they crank up your furnace to the max. From the moment your abdominal muscles engage to get you out of bed in the morning and your leg muscles contract as you walk to the kitchen, the energy you burn through physical activity accounts for 25 to 35 percent of your daily calories. This *thermic effect of physical activity*, or TEPA, accounts for all the energy you burn through muscle contractions.

Your muscles store only 5 to 10 seconds worth of energy , which is basically just enough to get you moving. When you continue moving, your muscles need more calories. Every time your body requires calories to function, your metabolism starts roaring, and you are on your way to losing weight. Following The Carb-Cycle Solution, you'll do *shredder* cardio exercises every day. These are specifically designed to spike your metabolic furnace to "blazing" for maximum fat loss. The more muscle you can develop and the more muscle you put into motion, the more calories you burn!

BODY SMARTS

Many people believe that because they've been overweight all their life or because they're overweight now, they won't be able to lose their excess pounds. Whenever you hear someone say, "I have a slow metabolism," you can share with him or her the four secrets of turning up their metabolic furnace for maximum weight loss. It isn't rocket science, just textbook physics and physiology!

Evolution equipped our bodies with a system of checks and balances that ensures survival in as many conditions as possible. Our ancestors often went hungry, so the body adapted to become much more efficient at using and conserving the calories coming in, and the body figured out something ingenious: If less energy (food) is coming in, then less energy (calories) should go out. Bottom line: When you eat fewer calories day after day, your body adjusts its metabolism to lose as little weight as possible. If you want to lose weight, you have to work with your body's metabolism.

The intelligence of your body and its ability to survive times of food scarcity is something to respect and celebrate. Thank goodness our bodies *can* adjust, or our prehistoric ancestors would not have survived, and we would not be here today.

THE TRUTH

Established principles determine how your body furnace burns calories, yet myths about weight loss abound. You may be surprised to find that some commonly held beliefs about weight loss are actually not true.

WEIGHT–LOSS **MYTHS & FACTS**

MYTHS	FACTS
All people who are overweight eat too much, too often.	Many overweight people eat too little, too infrequently.
If you eat a very low–calorie diet, you will easily reach your ideal weight.	Your body adapts to a low-calorie diet by lowering its metabolism, making it more difficult to lose weight.
You should eliminate one of the macronutrients (carbohydrates, proteins, or fats) from your diet to lose weight.	Your body is designed to use all three macronutrients. If you eliminate any of them, you undermine your health, metabolism, and weight loss.
Skipping meals and eating infrequently is the best way to lose weight.	You must eat frequently, and eat enough, to raise your metabolism. A high metabolism is key to weight loss.
Eating two to three meals a day is optinmal for weight loss.	Eating five smaller meals a day has been shown to be more effective than eating three meals a day for curbing cravings and preventing overeating.
It takes the same amount of calories to digest different kinds of food, no matter what you eat.	Digesting protein requires more calories than breaking down carbohydrates or fat. Eating protein helps boost your metabolism.
Muscle and fat burn the same amount of calories.	Muscle burns *many* more calories than fat, so the bigger your muscles, the higher your metabolism.
Eating less and exercising more will help raise your metabolism.	Eating enough of the right food frequently throughout the day will help raise your metabolism. Add exercise to boost your metabolism even more!
Cardiovascular exercise alone is the best way to work out to reach your weight-loss goals.	A combination of cardiovascular exercise and resistance training is the healthiest and fastest way to achieve optimal fitness.

Now that you understand the power of your metabolism, let's explore the power of your mind to transform your body.

CHAPTER 5:
CHANGE YOUR MIND, CHANGE YOUR BODY

"If you are going to win any battle you have to do one thing. You have to make the mind run the body. Never let the body tell the mind what to do. The body will always give up. It is always tired in the morning, noon and night. But the body is never tired if the mind is not tired."
—General George S. Patton, U.S. Army, 1912 Olympian

When you were born, you were given the most incredible gift you will ever receive—your body. All the other stuff you acquire in your lifetime—cars, houses, tools, toys—comes and goes, but your body will always be there. So without your physical health, you have nothing. There are three things you can do to reach optimum health by taking charge of your weight-loss transformation. You can learn to eat right. You can add the right kind of exercise to your lifestyle. But first of all, you must put your mind to work.

As you begin The Carb-Cycle Solution, you'll learn some amazing tricks to manipulate your body for maximum fat loss. Before you can do that, however, you must first uncover and discover who you really are, mentally and emotionally. My wish is for your weight loss to last a lifetime. My goal is for you to truly transform! To do so, you have to change your mind as well as your body.

YOU AND YOUR MACHINE

I can't tell you how many times I've heard people say that when they look in the mirror they see people who aren't *them*. They feel trapped in their unhealthy, overweight bodies, confined to a prison they don't deserve. Why? Because when we look in the mirror, we only see our physical body. We see a machine that has been handed down through generations of ancestors. And we see what we've done to it. We see the results of our lifestyle, not the essence of who we are as thinking, feeling, desiring people.

From the moment you were born—and for your entire time on earth—you and your machine will coexist. You can't choose another one. A harmonious connection between you and your machine can take you to untold heights. But if you try to work independently of each other, your machine will take over.

Your machine is the house for YOU: your soul, your being, your mind, your unique, magical spark of life. Your consciousness is the true you. You know what's good for you in the long run. You can reason. You have dreams and hopes. You can set goals for yourself. You *know* you should wake up early every day. You *know* you should eat healthy foods, and you *know* you should exercise for an hour every day. That's you—your mind—talking!

YOU MUST MASTER THE MACHINE

Your body, the machine, is primitive. It runs on instinct, driven by the mechanisms that have ensured its survival for thousands of years. If it's allowed to run free, your machine will eat as much food as is available. It has no limitations, no guidance. Your primitive machine probably wants to sleep in, eat junk food, and play video games all day. Its voice chatters in your head, talking you into bad habits and addictions even though your mind *knows* they aren't good for you.

Raw emotions fuel your machine. When you're happy, sad, frustrated, depressed, lonely, elated, or angry, it rationalizes, urging you to turn your emotions into bad habits and addictions. Because you're an emotional creature, your machine will challenge you for the rest of your life.

If you don't take control of your machine, it will eventually wreak havoc on itself—and you. As a thinking human being, you have the ability to control your machine. You have a mind! Your mind has goals, but you can't achieve them without your machine to put your plans into motion. To accomplish your dreams and aspirations, you must take charge of your machine and make it work for you.

To gain power over your machine, you must fight battles every day to complete your daily exercise and eat healthy instead of satisfying your cravings. Every time you do what you know is best for your health and happiness, you win a battle with your machine.

Each daily victory will build upon the last until you reach the point where your emotion-fueled machine is no match for you. When your machine submits to your mind, they work together in harmony . . . and are unstoppable. Together, you can accomplish anything and everything you set out to achieve, from breaking destructive habits to loosing as much weight as you need to!

KNOW YOUR MACHINE

When I first start working with clients, I put them through this exercise to help them gain a powerful awareness of the relationship between mind and body. At first they think it is pretty funny, but when they do it they see themselves from a whole new prespective! Stand in front of a mirror, shirt off, and follow these steps:

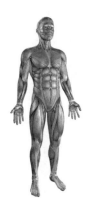

Underneath the skin and body fat, this is what we all look like.

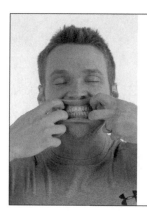

Pull back lips

Grab your lips and pull them back so you can see your jaw and teeth. *See* and picture the skull inside.

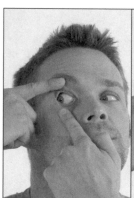
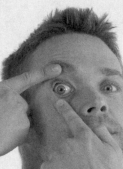
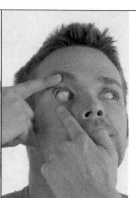

Pull back eyelids

Pull back your eyelids and *see* your eyeballs. *See* and imagine the nerves running from your eyeballs to your brain. Remember that the only reason you know you're standing in front of a mirror is that it's reflecting light that forms an image on the back of your eyeballs. Your eyeballs send the image to your brain that tells you, "I'm standing in front of a mirror."

Push skin on face

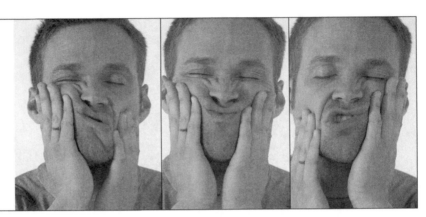

Now grab the skin on your face. Push it around. Play with it. Move your jaw. Feel the bone structure of the skull beneath. Really observe and experience your machine.

Grab your fat

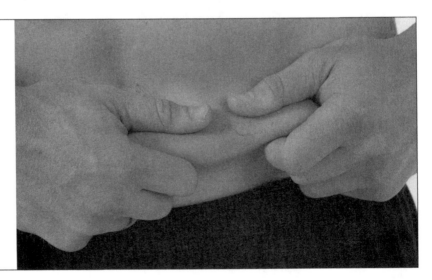

Move farther south and feel your abdomen. Feel the layer of body fat. Grab it. Squeeze it. While holding it, understand that your body fat is simply a layer of unused energy—that's all. It's a sign that your body is beautifully efficient. When you consume more calories than your body can burn, it does exactly what it's supposed to do: It stores those calories up for a leaner time when you might need extra energy. See your body fat for what it is. Appreciate it for the first time.

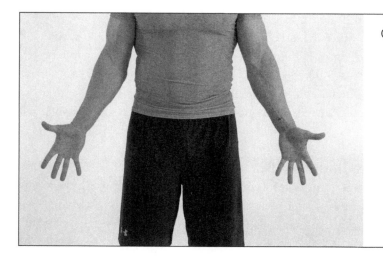

Open hands

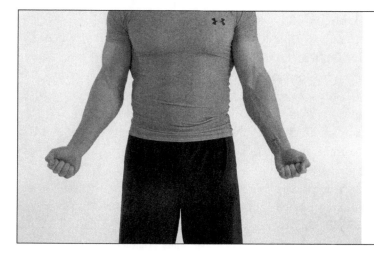

Close hands into fists

Watch your hands as they open and close. Examine them. Visualize the electrical signal running from your brain down your spinal cord, to the muscles that lengthen and contract to extend and flex your fingers. See the machine at work!

Now that you've glimpsed your machine of skin, bones, muscle, blood, and organs, name it. It's yours, your project, your pet. Name it anything you want.

The name of my body is: _____.

Remember, YOU are the mind. Your machine, your body, is at your command. Whether you want to lose 30 or 300 pounds, you can change your body. Walk it. Feed it. Water it. Rest it. Love it. Transform it.

You've named your machine and claimed ownership of it, so you, the mind, can now take control. The stronger your mind becomes through repeated victories over your machine, the easier it is to take charge, the faster you achieve your goals, and the better you feel about yourself!

If you didn't do the exercise, your machine is still in control. Take charge. Tell your machine what to do. Win a victory over your machine: Do the exercise!

INTEGRITY: COMMITMENT TO YOURSELF

At the start of your journey of transformation, you'll begin making daily commitments—promises—that you need to keep in order to reach your goal to be slim and healthy. Commit to eating five meals, drinking a gallon of water, and doing your resistance shapers and cardio shredder exercises every day. Some daily commitments may seem monotonous at first: Your machine won't want to do them and will find any reason not to. To empower yourself, however, it's imperative to fulfill the commitments you make.

True empowerment is rooted in something called integrity. When this principle is present in our lives, transformation becomes possible. If we choose to neglect this principle, transformation becomes impossible. So what is integrity? I have yet to come across a better definition than the one given by Stephen R. Covey in *The 7 Habits of Highly Effective People:*

"Integrity is, fundamentally, the value we place on ourselves. It's our ability to make and keep commitments to ourselves, to 'walk our talk.' It's honor with self, the essence of proactive growth."

To live with integrity is to honor your word and commitments, to yourself first, and then to others. By following through on your daily health commitments, you grow your own self-worth so that you can take greater and greater control of your machine. As this happens, you begin to see your potential to take on bigger challenges. Your machine is at your command. You start to see that your target is within reach.

SABOTAGING YOUR SELF-RESPECT

Living with integrity is a daily choice. Heck, it's an hourly choice. How many times have you promised yourself, "I'll start the diet on Monday," or "Tomorrow I'm going to wake up early to exercise." Sure enough, when the alarm goes off, your machine quickly comes up with a reason to sleep in. By noon on Monday, your machine rationalizes why it needs pizza and ice cream for dinner. At the end of the day, you feel like a complete failure.

You can concoct all the reasons and excuses in the world, like "I didn't get enough sleep last night so I needed to sleep in," or "I didn't have any other food available on Monday night," but the *fact* is that you've let yourself down. You've lost the battle with your machine. You've broken your promise to yourself, and you'll do all you can to hide your shame from others. Your self-esteem has taken yet another devastating blow. Sound familiar?

Day after day, week after week, month after month, year after year, promise after broken promise, you've fallen so deep into despair that it seems there's no more hope—until you make a simple declaration. It's time to be authentic with yourself . . . truly and completely honest.

Look into the mirror and say to yourself, "I have not fulfilled promises that I have made to myself. It has hurt my self-esteem and confidence. But now I am re-commiting to my goals!"

GROWING YOUR INTEGRITY

Right now, your integrity—the value you place on yourself—is delicate. It needs to be nurtured to grow. Reversing its decline begins by fulfilling just one small promise. One promise leads to two. Two leads to three, and so on.

Every silent promise fulfilled nourishes your self-respect a little bit more. You begin to believe your own promises again. Promise after promise fulfilled eventually builds your sense of self-worth to substantial proportions. What was once a weak and delicate seedling is now a towering redwood. When you set out to accomplish something—anything—it gets done.

When you're living with integrity, your mind is in harmony with your machine, and your self-esteem and confidence flourish. They grow every time the two parts of you share in victory together. Each triumph has a domino effect, triggering the next. You, the mind, set the daily goal, and your machine accomplishes it.

But don't take my word for it. You must *feel* it. I can't come close to describing the powerful effect growing your integrity will have on you. When my clients reach the end of their weight-loss journey and try to explain their newfound confidence and self-esteem, they can't. To fully understand how a full-grown sense of self-worth feels is to experience it for yourself.

EXPECTATIONS: THE LOTTERY SYNDROME

As the saying goes, "Disappointment is simply unmet expectations." Expectations can be double-edged swords. When expectations are met, they can motivate us to new heights, giving us the courage to try new things and take bold steps toward a greater future. However, when expectations are too grand and unmet, they can leave us feeling let down and frustrated—emotions that open the way for our machine to take control.

Soon after you set out on your Carb-Cycle Solution journey, you'll see results, and before you know it you'll reach your goal. But before you get going, let's dispel a myth about your weight-loss destination: Many of my transformation clients begin the process believing that when they reach that magic weight something glorious happens. Life is forever changed. Problems disappear. Life is smooth sailing from now on. But it isn't.

This the lottery syndrome. Despite their expectations, people who win the lottery quickly realize that their problems don't go away. They may be able to pay off their bills, but all their other issues continue to dog them. They don't find happiness in money.

I'm going to be honest with you: You won't find happiness when you reach your weight-loss goal. What you *will* discover is far greater. It transcends weight loss and permeates every aspect of your life. Along the path to your destination, you'll realize that when you fulfill your daily commitments, you become empowered in a way you never imagined. You become powerful, limitless.

The transformation process is where you'll find all the power, all the beauty, all the pride. Does the *process* lead to happiness? It certainly can—it's up to you! Your journey isn't about what you are at the end, but about whom you *become* along the way. When you, the mind, take control of your machine and the two of you work together in true harmony to overcome life's everyday obstacles, you'll be rewarded with a beautiful body, health, confidence, self-respect, and genuine happiness. Something magical happens when you meet your commitments to yourself and make your machine follow through with action. A silent promise is fulfilled.

Transformation is a lifetime commitment that you should be excited about! This isn't a short journey. Don't expect to grit your teeth and bear it for a few months, then go back to your old lifestyle. Transformation is for the rest of your life. The Carb-Cycle Solution can make it enjoyable, so you can be empowered one, five, ten years down the road!

FAILURE IN TWO WORDS

Two simple words can threaten your integrity, your commitment to yourself. At one time or another, most people who want to lose weight make a common blunder when they think about the challenges they face. Instead of committing to triumph in the battle between mind and machine, they say the two weakest words in the English language:

"I'll try."

When we're not prepared to truly make a commitment, we *try*. Saying "I'll try" means our soul isn't really in it. We tell ourselves "I'll try" when our inflated egos won't come clean and admit that we're actually not all that determined. We can't overcome obstacles with the words "I'll try." As Yoda, the philosopher in the *Star Wars* movies, says,

"Do, or do not. There is no 'try.'"

The choice to *do* is up to us. We might not be able to do the impossible, but we can achieve the unlikely. Meeting and conquering challenges is within our grasp. Every time we *do*, we make a leap. One success leads to the next, and before we know it, we've reached our goal. There may be bumps along the way, but each one teaches us something that allows us to progress toward our goal. Honor your commitment to yourself:

"Today I won't just aim for my goal. I'll take action to *reach* my goal."

FALL WITHOUT FAILING

"It's not about how many times you fall down, but how many times you get back up." —Abraham Lincoln

Even with obstacles in your way—perhaps *especially* with obstacles in your way—you can move confidently toward your weight-loss goal. Let's be honest: Life isn't fair. It's sometimes turbulent and harsh. Anything can and will happen. The only thing that's guaranteed is that you *will* be challenged. All kinds of curveballs will be thrown at you during your journey of transformation. That's real life. Troubles and roadblocks will always be around the next corner.

On your transformation journey, I can guarantee that you'll encounter challenges of your own, such as financial difficulties, relationship problems, work worries, or health issues. You'll experience a wide range of emotions along the way: elation, anger, sadness, disappointment, frustration, you name it. Bottom line: expect trouble to happen because it will. The question is, how will you react? Will emotions manipulate your machine enough to defeat you, destroying your self-respect and sending you into a downward spiral? Will you have the power and awareness to take control and win a major victory over your machine?

It's time to welcome life's challenges as your unique opportunity to grow stronger. Difficult times are the true proving ground for your most powerful mental tools: perseverance, resolve, and resourcefulness. You can find solutions to anything if you choose to. Make this declaration:

"From this moment on I will face each and every downfall in life as an opportunity to become stronger. I will use my resolve, perseverance, and resourcefulness to find solutions and meet my daily commitments."

ONE MORE SECRET: *BEING* WITH THE END IN MIND

There's a secret to giving your mind full control over your machine, making your transformation possible. Have you ever heard the saying "beginning with the end in mind?" To transform, to have the body you've always wanted, you must have not only a definite plan but also a clear, concise, vivid picture of what you want. Your goal is the end of your weight-loss journey.

Think about your goal. What will you look like? What will you feel like? What will success taste, smell, sound like? What will people say when they see you? Family and friends who haven't seen you in a while—how will they react? How will people treat you?

Let's visualize you at your goal. The clock goes off at 6 am and you turn off the alarm. You're still tired and slowly get out of bed. But something is different. You put your feet on the floor and realize that you've finished your weight-loss journey. Your body feels light. Your skin is tight against your muscles. You reach up and stretch, then scratch your belly, feeling the hard muscles of a tight six-pack. Your arms, stomach, and legs are lean and toned. You've reached your goal weight. What do you eat for breakfast? What do you do for exercise? Throughout the day, meal by meal, moment by moment, feel what it's going to be like to lead a transformed life.

How can this happen? I'm going to give you a hint: It begins with changing your sense of who you are. Start your transformation journey by *being* the person you want to be. *Be* that person now. Practice *being* with the end in mind.

WHO ARE YOU?

Take a look at your sense of identity. Are you strong willed and in control of your machine? Are you weak, so your machine takes over and does what it wants? What are you like in difficult situations, when life isn't fair? Is your mind powerful enough to stay the weight-loss course when times are tough, or does your machine take over?

How do you become strong enough to control your machine all the time? Believe it or not, your identity—the way you view yourself—is one of the biggest influences on the choices you make. Your identity has many facets, with one or two topmost for each of us. Explore these identities for yourself! Write down your own identities, and circle the ones that are most important to you.

Relationship Identity. Examples: I am a father; I am a daughter; I am a lover; I am a friend.

I am _____

Occupation Identity. Examples: I am an accountant; I am a homemaker; I am a lawyer; I am a computer technician.

I am _____

Sport/Hobby Identity. Examples: I am a gamer; I am a stamp collector; I am a musician; I am an athlete.

I am _____

Group/Origin Identity. Examples: I am a Christian; I am a Latino; I am a Westerner; I am an American.

I am _____

Physical Identity. Examples: I am fat; I am weak; I am tall; I am ill; I am strong.

I am _____

Emotional Identity. Examples: I am weak-willed; I am a coward; I am optimistic; I am a fighter.

I am _____

For better or worse, your identity is colored by what you think it means. Your sense of identity might be destructive:

"I don't do cardio. I've always been that way."

"I'm Southern, and Southerners eat fried food."

"I'm a New Yorker, and New Yorkers don't hike."

"I'm weak. I give in to my friends when they want to party."

Can't you hear these declarations of identity eroding and undermining your self-worth? They all say the same thing: "This is the way I am, and there's nothing that can change it." Controlling your decisions, thoughts like these crush your self-will when you face tough situations. You rationalize your defeatism by saying, "It's not my fault, it's who I am." In other words, your identity made you do it. It's one of the greatest lies you can tell yourself. If you choose to embrace a rigid and unchangeable identity, you're doomed to follow a pre-ordained path into an inevitable future. But there is hope. . . .

TAKE A LOOK AT YOURSELF

Who you *think* you are dictates how you react to situations you encounter daily. It determines whether you can put mind over machine. A simple exercise illustrates the point. It requires some imagination, but I challenge you to try it out and see how it feels.

Situation A

You've just been at an office party where you did a good job avoiding the buffet table loaded with mini corndogs, crab puffs, and potato chips. Leaving the office, you're starving. With no one there to see you, you turn onto a street of fast-food drive-throughs.

1. You are a strong-willed athlete-in-training. You're a winner. What do you do in this situation?

2. You are a weak-willed, overweight social reject. What do you do in this situation?

The food tastes the same to both people, but you can take a good guess at the outcome of the situation. Which person has more integrity, self-esteem, and confidence? Who's most likely to reach their goals and fulfill their aspirations? Which one do you want to be?

Situation B

The alarm goes off at 6 am. You've allocated an hour for exercise, but you didn't get to bed until midnight, and you're exhausted. Maybe you'll just sleep in.

1. You are a strong-willed athlete-in-training. You're a winner. What do you do in this situation?

2. You are a weak-willed, overweight, social reject. What do you do in this situation?

Both people are exhausted when the alarm goes off, but you can take a good guess at the outcome for each. Which person has more integrity, self-esteem, and confidence? Who's most likely to reach their goals and fulfill their aspirations? Which one do you want to be?

Get it? You'll always live according to your vision of your identity. How you view yourself is your future.

Even when you're totally ready to change, transformation can seem like a formidable undertaking. But you can choose an identity that makes you strong. If you identify yourself as someone who's fit, you'll want to make decisions that benefit your health and wellness. You'll want to choose the right foods at the grocery store, to do something active instead of sitting in front of that television show, to be strong when others tempt you with something that undermines your goal. When you become a person with a positive identity, you *live into* a better life.

As you can see, your identity can be beneficial or destructive. It's your sense of self, which guides you in your daily decisions. You can *choose* who you want to be. Once you realize that your identity can evolve, you empower yourself to take on and conquer any challenge in life.

A STRONG IDENTITY = SUCCESS

There's an athlete in all of us. Yes, there's an athlete in *you*! Take on this fitness identity, no matter how much fat weighs down your machine. *Be* an athlete-in-training. When any athlete begins training, they feel out of shape. But meal after meal, workout after workout, week after week, they build strength, stamina rises, endurance is enhanced, and the fat falls off. You have the capacity to become strong, lean, and powerful. Take on the fitness identity of an athlete, and live into it. Try it on, and see how it feels.

From this moment on, YOU ARE AN ATHLETE-IN-TRAINING. This is your fitness identity. For the first several weeks of your transformation, you need to practice feeling your fitness identity. It'll be all too easy to slip back into your old identity. Use a visual reminder if you need to. I use a permanent marker on my legs. Seriously!

This kind of change is powerful stuff. It's not easy. Not everybody is ready to explore a new identity that can change his or her life. You are whomever you choose to be. We're all free agents. We either do or don't allow our minds to control our machines.

Along the way on your transformation journey, you'll encounter life's obstacles and challenges. Some days you won't fulfill your commitments to yourself. But it's what you do next that matters. Do you give up, or do you recommit, choose to take on a stronger, winning identity, and start again?

Winners see problems as opportunities to gain insight and tough times as occasions for growth. If they begin a project, they finish it. Finishing your transformation will give you a better quality of life. Physically, you'll end up with less body fat, more muscle, and better stamina, to name a few benefits. Mentally, you'll have rebuilt your self-esteem, taken your integrity to new heights, and discovered your inner power to commit to and accomplish anything!

TOM'S STORY

Let me tell you about a good friend of mine whom I've worked with on my television show, *Extreme Makeover: Weight Loss Edition* on ABC. Tom once weighed 265 pounds, and when I first met him, he had already dropped to 200.

His weight-loss journey is the perfect example of the power of identity. Tom wrote to me, "Just a few short years ago, I weighed nearly 100 pounds more than I do today. I was overweight, lazy and self-loathing. I tried everything to lose the weight. I lost weight, I gained it back, I lost even more weight and I gained it all back again. I've struggled like most people to find something that worked for me and lasted more than a couple months. I hated exercising and I hated eating 'healthy.' Every time I looked in the mirror, I hated the body that was looking back at me. I felt lost."

Tom said he wanted to reach a new level of fitness and get into endurance sports. He wanted to compete in triathlons, to sequentially swim, cycle, and run to victory. He bought all the gear and started hanging out with a triathlete club.

"Weight started to come off as I found my identity. I had something that I could be proud of and something that defined who I was. I didn't even know how to swim but I'd be damned if I was going to let that stop me. I started running and had someone teach me how to swim. It was a struggle once again to get started but after weeks of practice, I finally was ready to take the leap."

Now, Tom has already participated in a handful of triathlons and is preparing for his first half-Ironman, a long-distance triathlon. Down to 170 pounds, his body—his machine—now reflects the person who was hiding under 265 pounds just a couple short years ago. Tom found an identity as a triathlete. Because he changed his identity, he changed his life.

"When I completed my first triathlon in January 2010, although I felt like one before, I was now able to officially call myself a TRIATHLETE. What an amazing feeling that was. I felt powerful and I realized that I could do anything I set my mind to. I've completed four triathlons now and have set my next goal to complete the Vineman Half Ironman. I never thought this was possible a few years ago when I was that struggling, lazy, overweight person who didn't know who I was. I'm thankful that now, I do know. I am a triathlete."

CHAPTER 6:
ARE YOU READY?

As the saying goes, "Rock bottom is where you stop digging." If you've read this far, you've stopped digging and are clearly ready for a change. You've devoted time and energy to educating yourself about weight loss. You may have experienced a few moments of clarity that have triggered your desire to change. Perhaps you recently saw a picture of yourself and were unhappy with your appearance. Perhaps you can't fit into your favorite jeans anymore. Perhaps you feel like you're missing out on important relationships because you don't feel good about yourself. Perhaps you're too embarrassed to take your shirt off at the beach. Perhaps your doctor that has given you a wake-up call in the form of a serious diagnosis. You realize that the body of your dreams is finally within reach.

If you continue to follow your current lifestyle, how will your body look and feel five years from now? Ten years? Thirty years? Are you unintentionally shortening your lifespan? How will the quality of your life, not just the duration, be affected? Will you miss out on having fun with the people you love because you're overweight and out of shape? Will they be forced to care for you because you can't care for yourself? You can foresee the inevitable future you're creating for yourself.

Change will happen when life as you know it is so physically or emotionally painful that you can't imagine living another day as you are. Whether you are 30 or 300 pounds overweight, you vow never to live another day in your predicament. Some call this rock bottom. I call it rebirth. Rock bottom is different for everyone and is the pivotal point at which you take control of your destiny and search for solutions. Well, look no further. The Carb-Cycle Solution is here.

A wise person once said, "It is never too late to become who you might have been." You have the power to change, starting today.

ACTION CONQUERS FEAR

Your choice to change must come from deep emotional desire. When your current situation and habits are no longer worthwhile, you're moved to take action. Once you contemplate how you've lived your life up to this moment, you'll realize that by shedding excess fat you'll be able to live a longer, happier, healthier, more energized life. You realize that your old lifestyle patterns aren't working, and there are new possibilities for your life just around the corner.

But let's be honest: You're a creature of habit who's followed the same lifestyle patterns day in and day out for years. Those old lifestyle patterns are your safe place. You feel comfortable there. And here you are, deciding to change those patterns, to leave your safe place. You must step outside your comfort zone and try new things if you're going to have the healthy body, mind, and soul you desire.

This moment of clarity is powerful. It spurs you to look for answers, for some guidance in making the change you crave. I am absolutely confident that when you reach your goals and look back, you'll agree that making this choice is one of the best things you've ever done for yourself. It's a fun and awesome awakening! Are you ready?

I invite you to stop reading for a moment. Reflect on the importance of committing to this next phase of your life. There's no rush—this is a big decision. Take the time you need to consider life as it has been up to this moment, what you want it to be from now on, and what you're willing to do about it.

CALL TO ACTION

I ask all my transformation clients to begin their journey with a declaration:

"My current lifestyle is not working for me. I am ready for a change. I *choose* to use my inner strength and resourcefulness to fulfill the daily commitments that will lead to a thinner, healthier, happier me. I am now an athlete-in-training."

This isn't a silent promise—that's too easily broken. Say it out loud with conviction, preferably in front of others. Once you verbalize your feelings and commitments, you take responsibility. Don't read this book sitting on the sidelines and observing. Get in the game. If you're ready for a change, say it out loud, and mean it!

I'm honored that you'll be joining me on this life-transforming adventure. Remember, you don't have to worry about *how* you'll lose weight, because I'll be there every step of the way. Your body will become what it's designed to be: fit, strong, healthy, and beautiful. More importantly, your mind will gain the power and knowledge to control your body for the rest of your life. You're truly on the brink of an awesome new you.

Now let's get started!

CHAPTER 7:
GET *SMART*

Your weight-loss adventure has begun. As you embark on the journey, it's imperative to have a forceful, proactive plan—a well thought-out, consistent action strategy. It's time to go forward. Pull out a pen, and get ready to write down your SMART tactics.

FIVE SMART FUNDAMENTALS

To be successful, your weight-loss plan must meet five distinct criteria:

1. It must be *specific*. What exactly is your goal? Where do you want to go on this journey? A specific commitment, for example, is "My goal is to lose 45 pounds," or "My goal is to be a size six," or "My goal is to reduce my blood pressure to 120/80 and get my cholesterol under 200." Avoid generalizations like "I want to lose weight," or "I want to be healthy," or "I want to look good in the mirror." Don't get me wrong—those are good goals, but they aren't nearly specific enough, and they give your machine too much wiggle room.

Every journey has a starting line and a finishing line. If you only have a vague, generalized goal, you give your machine permission to move the finish line whenever it gets tired or the journey becomes difficult. You'll never build the character to win. You'll never reach your true goal, and deep down inside you'll hate yourself for it. Remember, integrity is built on setting and fulfilling specific commitments. Don't give in. You're the master. Tell your body where you want it to go:

My specific transformation goal is _____

_____

_____

_____

2. Your weight-loss plan must be *measurable*. You must be able to quantify your goal to make darn sure that you hit it. Don't evaluate your progress according to compliments from others or by subjective feedback, such as the way you look in the mirror. Set your precise weight-loss and health goals via one or more of the following:

Desired weight in pounds/kilograms _____

Desired fit in clothing size _____

Desired measurements in inches/centimeters

     Neck   _____

     Chest   _____

     Waist   _____

     Hips   _____

     Thigh   _____

Desired medical test results (blood panel, lipid profile, blood pressure, glucose tolerance, etc.) _____

_____

_____

I recommend that before you start The Carb-Cycle Solution program, you take a few minutes to measure your body. Just weeks or months from now (depending on how much weight you want to lose), you'll be so glad you did. When you're satisfied with the body you've sculpted through the program, take your measurements again. Seeing the difference in the numbers is absolutely exhilarating. Follow the instructions below, and keep this record in a safe place so you're sure to find it again.

Date: _____

Weight: _____

Clothing size: _____

Circumference Measurements:

Neck Measure the circumference of your neck at the midpoint, around the Adam's apple.

_____ inches

Chest Measure the circumference of your chest along the "nipple line." It's important to keep your arms at your side.

_____ inches

Waist Measure the circumference of your waist at the narrowest point (usually at the navel).

_____ inches

Hips Measure the circumference of your hips at the widest point (usually about 6 to 8 inches below your waist).

_____ inches

Thigh Measure the circumference of your RIGHT thigh at a point about 8 inches above the knee.

_____ inches

Put this information in a safe place so you can look at it after you've reached your fitness goal. When you compare your before and after measurements, you'll be so proud of yourself!

3. Your weight-loss goal must be *attainable*. It must line up with what you're willing and able to do every day to reach it. If achieving your goal requires five hours of time and energy a day, but you're a single mother working a full-time job, it's a good idea to reassess your target, and set a realistic goal that entails perhaps 30 minutes to an hour daily. If your goal requires the purchase of expensive equipment, but you're unemployed, you need to reconsider. On your journey, you must be resourceful with your time, energy, and money, so it's important to establish attainable goals that fit your situation.

What will make my goal attainable? _____

_____

_____

4. Your weight-loss plan must be *realistic*. It's not realistic, for instance, to lose 200 pounds in three months. If you try with high hopes to attempt this feat, I can assure you that you'll be sorely disappointed. Disappointment can put your journey in jeopardy by giving your emotion-driven machine a window of opportunity for sabotage. If you're on a 300-pound weight-loss journey, give yourself time. It can take up to two years. Your goal could be, "I will lose 300 pounds by today's date, two years from now." If you're looking to lose 30 pounds, you're more likely on a three-month journey. Your goal commitment could be, "I will be 30 pounds lighter in three months."

Realistic goals go hand-in-hand with attainable goals. Set goals that you know you're physically capable of achieving and truly believe are reachable. Your goals should fit into your lifestyle (with some reasonable lifestyle changes). One of the best ways to set a realistic goal is to see what others have done in situations similar to yours. Check out my Web site, www.chrispowell.com, for inspiration. If they can do it, so can you!

A great rule of thumb for estimating the amount of weight you can reasonably lose weekly is to take your current weight and divide it by 100. The number will give you an approximation of the amount of weight you can lose safely every week. For example, I weigh 185 pounds, so I can lose 1.85 pounds safely every week. However, this is a very rough estimate, and The Carb-Cycle Solution often delivers much greater weekly weight losses—sometimes up to double the expected amount.

What's a realistic weight-loss goal for me? _____

_____

_____

5. Your weight-loss plan must be *time-sensitive*. When you set a goal, you need to create a sense of urgency because getting there is important for your health and happiness. "Someday" isn't a destination. It gives your machine too much room to make excuses for procrastination and lapses. Excuses—explanations why it's OK to stray from your path—erode your promises to yourself. You can't commit to your weight-loss goal with the pledge "I'll get there eventually." Without a deadline, you won't. Give yourself a crystal-clear timeframe for weight loss.

I choose to reach my goal by the following date: _____

REMEMBER THE RULE

Sticking to these principles makes it easy to set yourself on the right course. And throughout your journey, it's easy to remind yourself of the keys to success. Any time you lose your way, remember that your weight-loss goal must be:

Specific

   Measurable

      Attainable

         Realistic

            Time-Sensitive

Taken together, these attributes make your plan SMART.

CHAPTER 8:
PREPARE FOR SUCCESS

One of my transformation mottos is "Success doesn't just happen. It's a result of the four Ps of action: Planning, Preparation, Performance, and Perseverance." Now that you've made your SMART *plan* for weight loss, the next step is to *prepare* for success. With the right preparation, you CAN win this battle! You have to set up your surroundings to be weight-loss-friendly because it's impossible to lose weight in an atmosphere filled with temptation instead of reinforcement. Replacing negative influences with positive influences is essential to your success.

Your life has been filled with enticements to gain weight. Everything about your surroundings has reinforced your old identity. But when you re-create your identity, you can start to look honestly at bad influences and make some choices.

Accessing your very real inner power—putting your mind in control of your machine—allows you to make good weight-loss choices. These choices make it possible to become a healthier, happier you. You must make the right choices when you shop for food, when you're tempted to watch TV instead of exercising, and when someone you know tempts you to do something that undermines your goal. I promise you that wise choices feel ten times better than the lazier alternatives.

You have the power to choose a healthy lifestyle. Once you do, you need to do everything you can to ensure you won't fail. Give your surroundings a face-lift to maximize your odds. Here's how to create an environment for success.

STOCK UP

If you surround yourself with influences that support your Carb-Cycle Solution goals, you are much more likely to stick with the program and achieve long-term success. Weight loss starts with nutrition, and nutrition starts in the grocery store. So you've got to stock up on food that will help you lose weight.

When I go grocery shopping, I remind myself as I pass by all the unhealthy foods that in the big picture they simply aren't worth it. I know that if I take them home, I'm more likely to eat them when I shouldn't. It's more important to me to be fit and healthy than to satisfy a craving for something that's bad for me. That's why I make a beeline for the protein and produce sections.

Do anything it takes to keep your fitness identity high and your temptations low when you get to the store, at least until buying good food becomes a habit. Many of my clients bring along a magazine picture of the body they'd like to have, just to reinforce their fitness identity in the grocery store!

A wonderful nutrition rule of thumb is not to shop on an empty stomach. It's a no-brainer: Cravings bother you less when you've got something in your stomach, so it's easier to make sensible and rational nutrition decisions.

When it comes to finding the best food in the supermarket, follow this simple and time-honored tip: Stay along the outside perimeter of the store. This is generally where you'll find the fresh meat, seafood, produce, and dairy sections. In addition, a couple aisles in the middle of the store—those with canned and frozen vegetables and fruit, dried herbs and spices, and other raw materials—are free of most pitfalls. With few exceptions, these are the only spots you need to hit when shopping for food. Turn to Chapter 9 for the Master Grocery List of approved foods. Find what you like, and stock up!

CLEAN OUT

When you get home from the store, you'll need a place to store all that healthy food. In order to make room—but more importantly, to give your weight-loss plan a fighting chance—throw out, or preferably donate, all the food in your house that will threaten your success. To donate your food, please visit www.feedingamerica.com, and search for a food bank near you. What better way to start your journey than by paying it forward to someone who needs the food?

I don't care if you have plenty of room for all your junk food as well as the healthy food: Get rid of the junk. If it's in your house, you're very likely to eat it. Why give your machine the opportunity to sabotage your progress? If those candy bars aren't on the shelf when you crave them, you can win an incredible victory over your machine. At the end of the day, you'll be glad you didn't eat the junk, and you'll be that much stronger. After a few weeks, when you've lost many pounds, you'll be glad you chose to dump the junk.

Foods to remove:

- Baked goods

- Beer

- Candy

- Chips

- Chocolate

- Conventional white and wheat breads

- Cookies

- Crackers

- Fried foods

- Frozen meals

- Hard alcohol

- Juice

- Ice cream

- Soda

- Wine

Also remove all foods containing the following ingredients:

- Brown sugar

- Corn syrup

- Honey

- Hydrogenated oils

- Maple syrup

- Raw sugar

- White flour

- White rice

- White sugar

On The Carb-Cycle Solution, you *will* be allowed to eat your favorite foods, but keeping them at home isn't a good idea. When you do eat them, do it outside the house, and don't take them home!

By filling your kitchen with healthy food and getting rid of the junk, you do yourself a huge favor: You prove you're serious about getting into shape. We all need support to reach our goals, and the most important support comes from yourself. You're quite literally offering yourself support by making your kitchen an environment for success.

VISUALIZE SUCCESS

If you know where you want to go, you know which direction to take. In your mind's eye, you can see your goal: the beautiful, sculpted body you've always wanted. Visual reminders of your goal can keep you on course and be powerful motivators. Pictures—of your dream body, the love of your life, your children, or anything else important to you—will help you stay on track. Find a picture of whatever motivates you to get fit, and put it everywhere: in the car, on your bathroom mirror, heck, even in the refrigerator! At least once a day, and every time you need a boost, spend time looking at that picture to reaffirm your commitment to yourself. We all have moments when we think, "Why am I doing this?" At those times, use your picture to remind yourself why you're pursuing transformation. You deserve a healthy, fit body, and you know your life will be better for it.

RALLY THE TEAM

No man is an island. We are not designed to go through life alone. Humans work together. We need a team, a tribe, a support system to survive. When we work together in harmony, we can accomplish so much more!

However, when we embark on a life-changing program, we need to look at individuals in our everyday lives and understand whether they are going to help and support us or possibly sabotage our progress. Their journey may not be yours, and in fact, they may have a different objective altogether, so it will be important to recognize which people in your life have goals that align with yours.

Research has proven that our social group is one of the most important factors in our weight. A thirty-two-year-long study published in the New England Journal of Medicine found that obesity actually spread in clusters among friends, spouses, siblings, and neighbors. A person's chance of becoming obese was actually greater if their friends were obese (57 percent more likely) than if they were genetically predisposed to obesity: a person with an obese sibling was only 40 percent more likely to become obese. This shows the nature of our innate need for social acceptance and the powerful role of the support system in influencing our choices.

FAMILY AND FRIENDS

Most people think that family and friends are the most important support system we can have. True: If they are onboard then your chances of success skyrocket. However, let's get real. Do not expect everyone to embrace change wholeheartedly. Some families and friends are not ready to make a transition to new lifestyle patterns, and feelings of resentment can arise if new ways are forced on them. When this happens, you may experience feeling segregated, feeling as if you are going against the group, and feeling cast out of social events.

RELATIONSHIPS (SPOUSES AND PARTNERS)

The relationship dynamic is certainly complicated. When partners support one another unconditionally, the possibilities for change are limitless. However, it is completely natural and human to worry about change. Sometimes, one partner worries about the other changing his or her physical appearance and leaving to find someone "better." At the start, it's vital to have an honest conversation with your partner to open up communication about any concerns or hesitations he or she may have about your transformation. Remember, this is a choice that YOU have made, but we must be aware that other individuals are affected by this change as well, and we need to be conscious of how they may react to the change in their lives. Let them know that this is a choice you have made and you'd like to speak openly and honestly with them so that it doesn't create issues for you both along the way.

From my experience, the spouses and partners who embark upon the journey and embrace the change along with their significant other take their relationship to a whole new level, exploring a deeper sense of appreciation and love for one another. However, your partner has a say in his or her own life, so give them the opportunity to either embrace this change or continue their regular ways.

Identify these characters in your support team:

The Teammate	Jumps in the game right next to you. Embraces the new lifestyle wholeheartedly and lives it with you.
The Fan	Supports and cheers you on from the sidelines, but isn't quite ready to make lifestyle changes themselves.
The Coach	Understands the hardships of the journey and gives guidance along the way.

Identify these characters to watch for:

The Pusher   Pushes comfort food on you out of love or concern, but makes you feel guilty if you refuse the offering.

The Competitor   Can be jealous or competitive and tries to one-up you whenever possible. May start a weight-loss regimen as well, but will not invite you to join. The Competitor may also try to test your will, so beware!

The Saboteur   Claims to support your weight loss journey but complains about the inconvenience of your new lifestyle. They may create some sort of distraction or argument when it is your time for food or exercise, or nag you to lighten up, encouraging unwanted behavior and bringing restricted foods into the house or workplace.

Remember, there is no right or wrong in this. Most likely the Pusher, Competitor, and Saboteur do not have malicious intentions. They just don't know of life any other way. They are dealing with their own issues. Everyone has their own vote in this. Don't dislike or carry resentment toward the people around you for the choices that they make, just understand them and identify the role they play in your journey, and then plan your own tactics accordingly. Look to surround yourself with a support team that will encourage you, and let nothing get in YOUR way!

If you are unable to find the support you need from family and friends, one of the best places to find a support system is at Overeaters Anonymous meetings or at one of your local gyms or recreation centers. There you will find like-minded active people who are embarking on the journey together. There are also many online support groups and chat rooms, both local and national, where you can get the emotional support you need and ask questions of others who have been on the journey or are currently going through it.

REARRANGE THE FURNITURE

It can be difficult to take on a fitness identity when your surroundings remind you of the old you. From the moment you wake up to the moment you go to sleep, your physical environment transmits stories, memories, and experiences of the old you. One of the most powerful mental tools you can use to reinforce your fitness identity is to rearrange the furniture in your house. It signifies your rebirth and the arrival of the new you. When you wake up in a bed that's against a different wall, or walk into your living room and sit in a chair where the sofa used to be, your new physical environment will reinforce your new fitness identity. Go ahead—try it!

TRIGGERS AND TACTICS

Knowledge is power, especially when it comes to understanding how you react in situations and how your emotions influence your choices in life. As creatures of habit, we tend to follow similar daily patterns and react in predictable ways to our environment. Triggers can cause us to react in ways that work against our goals.

Triggers are typically people or events/situations that elicit strong emotional reactions. We all have them. People triggers can arise from interaction with a spouse or partner, parent, son or daughter, sibling, in-laws, boss, bully, etc. Event triggers can be anything from deadlines at work, driving by the fast food joint, social gatherings, divorce or break-ups, winning a competition, going to a restaurant or movie, or even sitting down to watch TV at night. We can encounter these triggers anywhere or everywhere, on an hourly, daily, weekly basis, and monthly basis, and especially during the holidays.

When we enounter triggers, strong emotions come up—so strong that we feel the need for something to make us feel better, some kind of satisfaction to help cope with the situation. For many of us, this comes in the form of food. Does the trigger make you upset? Food makes you feel better. Frustrated? Food makes you feel better. Happy? Food makes you feel even better! However, we know that this is far from the truth. In fact, the wrong food and the wrong amount make us feel worse—both physically and emotionally.

Triggers are an incredible opportunity to learn about ourselves. They actually have nothing to do with the person or event in question, but spotlight areas of our life where we are out of control and our emotions take over. The emotions we feel from people triggers typically stem from our own unmet needs. Perhaps it is the need to feel understood or trusted. Maybe it is the desire to feel independent or safe. In any event, these needs are very important to us—so important that if we feel they are not met, the emotion-driven machine takes over. To take control of our bodies for good, we must be able to identify the triggers in our life and how we react to them, otherwise they will control us.

Can we embrace these triggers and work around them on our weight loss journey? Absolutely. We just need to be able to identify them first, then use tactics to cope with the situation. Remember that we will encounter triggers for the rest of our lives and these tactics can be used to remain in control and keep us marching toward our destiny as happier, healthier humans.

Certain tactics remain essential when dealing with triggers. The key is to snap your mind out of the "red zone" before your emotions go on autopilot. We want to hit your trigger experience from every angle that we can to get it under control.

We can use single or multiple tactics:

> *Teamwork*: Telling someone you trust about the feelings you are experiencing. This is the most powerful method to putting you in control.

> *Avoidance*: Staying away from the trigger situation until new habits and patterns are engrained.

> *Planning*: Anticipating and strategizing creative methods to reduce the emotional impact of the trigger.

> *Creating an Environment for Success:* Removing unwanted foods from the environment and surrounding yourself with visual reminders of what motivates you.

> *Distraction*: Keeping your mind occupied so there isn't time or room for the trigger to affect you.

> *Substitution*: Switching to a similar but less harm-producing item.

> *Tricking Your Mind*: Choosing a preplanned amount rather than an unlimited one.

> *Tricking Your Taste Buds*: Overwhelming your taste buds with taste sensations that remove desire for food.

Take your time looking through the lists of triggers below. Identify your triggers and keep an eye out for them in the near future. They are certain to arise! When they do, employ one or more of the trigger tactics to take control. It can be as simple as that.

TRIGGER: FOOD

If you find specific foods trigger binge behavior, use these tactics to beat the binge.

1 Teamwork: Call or text someone you trust and tell them how you are feeling.
2 Create an Environment for Success: Clear out all trigger foods from your home and workplace.
3 Avoid: For some people, certain foods are such strong triggers that they need to avoid these foods forever. However, for most, avoidance is a great tactic to practice for just several weeks or months as you learn new daily patterns for living happily without the trigger foods.
4 Substitute: Simply substitute one of the thousands of similar sweet or salty foods available for the specific trigger food. It is usually necessary to avoid only the specific trigger food.
5 Plan: Schedule specific meals during the week to reward yourself with foods you enjoy.
6 Trick Your Mind: Get pre-portioned and packaged cheat-day foods. This will give your body the taste it desires, but stops you after finishing the portion-controlled package.

TRIGGER: INTERACTION WITH ANOTHER PERSON(S)

Understand that you cannot change the other person or the situation. It's very important to recognize your feelings by identifying specific emotions that are coming up and understanding that the desire to eat stems from basic needs that you feel are unmet. Examples: the need to feel understood, the need to feel trusted, the need to feel safe, the need to feel independent, and so on.

1 Teamwork: Tell someone you trust (a teammate!) about your emotions and desire to turn to food. This is the most powerful method to put you in control.

TRIGGER: BOREDOM

Boredom never leads to anything good, especially when it comes to food. I call the result "hypno-bingeing," since most bored eaters rarely remember their actions—it's as if they were hypnotized when eating. They can open a bag of chips, and when they finally snap out of the trance, the bag is gone. If you find yourself bored and wandering to the pantry or fridge, then try these tactics to battle the hypno-binge.

1. Teamwork: Call or text someone you trust and tell them how you are feeling.
2. Create an Environment for Success: Place a picture of your motivation in the cupboard, refrigerator, or wherever you find yourself snacking.
3. Plan: Get all junk foods out of the house! If they are in the house, you will eat them.
4. Substitute: Have healthy low-calorie snacks and drinks available.
5. Distract: Make yourself busy. Do something that you are passionate about. Pick up a hobby or start a project that you are excited about and will keep you busy.
6. Trick Your Mind: Have only prepackaged portion-sized amounts on hand.
7. Trick Your Taste Buds: Between meals, brush your teeth, chew mint gum, or suck on a strong breath mint.

TRIGGER: FAST FOOD DRIVE-THRU

If you cannot seem to drive past your local fast food joint without stopping for a fix, then use these tactics to defeat the drive-thru.

1. Teamwork: Call or text someone you trust and tell them how you are feeling.
2. Create an Environment for Success: Place a picture of your motivation on the dashboard to remind you why you are embracing a healthy lifestyle.
3. Avoid: Find an alternate route to avoid the temptation.
4. Plan: Prepare and carry food and water with you, so you're never hungry.
5. Trick Your Taste Buds: Keep mint gum or strong breath mints available to shock your taste buds if cravings get strong.

TRIGGER: GOING TO A RESTAURANT

Many people consider eating out a time to splurge. However, if restaurants are a part of your regular weekly routine, this mindset can set you up for disaster. Use these tactics to resist the restaurant rampage.

1   Teamwork: Call or text someone you trust and tell them how you are feeling.

2   Avoid: Stay away from any bread, chips, nuts, alcoholic beverages, etc. before the meal.

3   Plan: Split your entrée with your dining partner.

4   Plan: Have the waiter bring a to-go bag with your meal and split your portion immediately (or request they split it in the kitchen): half on your plate, half to take home.

5   Substitute: Order from the appetizer section to keep portions reasonable.

6   Substitute: Order baked, steamed, grilled, or boiled entrees instead of fried or sautéed entrees.

7   Trick the Taste Buds: Always order sauces and dressings on the side. Typically the flavor of the meal is enough. If not, with sauces on the side, you control the amount of added calories poured onto the meal.

TRIGGER: GOING TO THE MOVIES

Find yourself craving popcorn and candy every time you go to the movies? Use these tactics to take control and master the movie going experience.

1   Plan: Eat or take a fiber supplement beforehand to feel full.

2   Substitute: Get a low-calorie or calorie-free sweetened beverage.

3   Trick the Taste Buds: Bring mint-flavored gum.

TRIGGER: SOCIAL GATHERINGS

Find yourself itching to nibble with your friends in social situations? Use these tactics to beat the buffet.

1 Teamwork: Call or text someone you trust and tell them how you are feeling. Perhaps invite them to the event if possible.

2 Plan: Eat or take a fiber supplement beforehand to feel full.

3 Avoid: If possible, avoid the areas where the food is available.

4 Substitute: Bring your own healthy foods.

5 Substitute: Keep your hands full: Grab a low-calorie or calorie-free drink as soon as you get there. Continue holding a drink the whole time to keep your hands occupied.

6 Trick the Taste Buds: Start chewing mint-flavored gum before you even walk in the door.

TRIGGER: THE WORKPLACE

Find yourself yearning for junk food when dealing with the daily grind at work? An abusive boss or crass co-workers can certainly take an emotional toll. Use these tactics to win control over your workplace.

1 Teamwork: Call or text someone you trust and tell them how you are feeling.

2 Create an Environment for Success: Clean out any and all junk food from the office cupboards and your desk drawers.

3 Plan: Prepare and pack your food to bring with you.

4 Avoidance: Avoid the areas of the office where you feel tempted (donuts near the coffeemaker, vending machines, cafeteria, etc.).

Identify the triggers that you experience in your everyday life. What are they?

People Triggers: _____

_____

_____

_____

_____

_____

_____

Event/Situation Triggers: _____
_____
_____
_____
_____
_____
_____

NOW'S THE TIME

You've prepared your mind, your life, and your body for success, and it's time to embark on your journey. The path may be rough at times, but I'll guide you every step of the way to help you lose the weight you want to drop and to gain the fitness you seek.

Congratulations on your decision to transform your life. Let The Carb-Cycle Solution begin!

PART TWO:
ACTION

CHAPTER 9:

THE CARB-CYCLE SOLUTION: THE 7-DAY CARB CYCLE

Welcome to The Carb-Cycle Solution! I've fine-tuned this system over the past decade and have seen countless clients create their own success stories, from shred-downs that sculpt average folks into beach-ready bodies to 400-pound weight-loss transformations of the super-overweight. In my television show, *Extreme Makeover: Weight Loss Edition* on ABC, I share the stories of incredible transformations by some of my obese clients. Their epic journeys are so inspiring. If they can do it, so can you!

To pump up your own inspiration, visit www.chrispowell.com to see what my work is all about. The Carb-Cycle Solution can help you lose as much weight as you want and will show you how to avoid gaining the weight back. After following the plan laid out for you in this book, you'll look at weight loss and how it's accomplished with new eyes. What seemed to be an unattainable goal, perhaps never to be realized, will become simple, possible, and ultimately real.

You'll feel better and have far more energy. When you look in the mirror, you'll see a new and beautiful you—the physical body you've always wanted to have. You'll know exactly how you got there and why it worked. You'll know how to make smart choices about your lifestyle and how your weight will be affected by those choices for the rest of your life.

With The Carb-Cycle Solution:

- You'll learn how to control your body to shed weight and body fat.
- You'll feel your body changing as it reacts to the program.
- You'll eat the foods you crave.
- You'll build lean, strong muscles.

• You'll increase your endurance, stamina, and cardiovascular health.

• You'll conquer the dieter's plateau.

WHAT IS CARB CYCLING?

The Carb-Cycle Solution plan is broken down into one-week segments. Each 7-Day Carb Cycle uses the power of a process called *carbohydrate cycling*. Carbohydrate cycling is a secret weapon in the health and fitness industry, used for over thirty years to maximize fat loss while maintaining muscle. The Carb-Cycle Solution takes carbohydrate cycling to a whole new level and puts a real-life twist on it.

Carb cycling for weight loss is easy: Eat meals that are high in carbohydrates every other day. Eat meals that are low in carbohydrates on the days in between. It's as simple as that. However, each 7-Day Carb Cycle also cycles your *calories* on high- and low-carbohydrate days, to amp up your fat loss. The back and forth between high-calorie/high-carb days and low-calorie/low-carb days revs your metabolic furnace and makes your body *think* it's eating enough on low days so it keeps burning calories. Just when you've completed a high-carb/high-calorie day, and your body is convinced there's no reason to be stingy by lowering your metabolism, you follow it with a low-carb/low-calorie day when you burn fat.

The meals and portions in each 7-Day Carb Cycle (see Chapter 15) are designed to cycle your carbohydrates and calories, so just follow the plan and carb cycle away!

WHY CYCLE CARBS?

Your body is never static. It conducts a symphony of metabolic reactions every moment. As your metabolic furnace burns (either on low heat or red-hot) every minute of every day, nutrients are constantly shuttled into or out of your muscle and fat cells to be stored or used as fuel for the critical metabolic reactions that keep you alive.

On high-carb/high-calorie days, your body is predominantly in what's called an *anabolic* state. The term *anabolic* describes periods when nutrients are being transferred into your cells, and you're in a state of building up. When your body's breaking down fat tissue to fuel your cells (on your low-carb/low-calorie days) it's in a *catabolic* state. To achieve fat loss, you want most of the fuel burned by your body to come from your fat cells. So you want to be catabolic most of the time!

Now, keep in mind that you don't want to be catabolic *all* the time. Both the anabolic and catabolic states have their beauty. In an anabolic state, you're building muscle and turning up your metabolic thermostat: Your muscle furnace burns hotter. When you're catabolic, your metabolic thermostat gets turned down. Your muscle furnace slowly cools off, but with The Carb-Cycle Solution you're burning fat at a rapid rate!

What if you could control your furnace's on and off switch? Believe it or not, you can. Yes, you can! YOU control when you build muscle and boost your metabolic rate and when you burn fat. Control the switch and you control your body.

How? With carb cycling, of course! Carbohydrates are anabolic foods: When they break down into glucose, your body triggers the hormone insulin to drive nutrients into your cells. During this process, your metabolic thermostat gets turned up. So what happens when you stop eating carbs? Your body switches into a predominantly catabolic state, maximizing the mobilization and burning of fat for fuel.

Are you starting to see the beauty of carb cycling? When you consume carbs on one day, you drive nutrients into your cells, building muscle and revving up your metabolic furnace. The next day you cut your carbs, essentially flipping the switch to turn your body into a prime-time fat-burning furnace!

WHY CYCLE CALORIES?

From day to day, each 7-Day Carb Cycle cycles calories as well as carbs. Changing your calorie intake on alternating days prevents your body from adapting and slowing weight loss. It forces your body to boost its metabolism one day, and then mobilize and burn fat stores the next. By cycling carbs this way, your body is more likely to avoid the dreaded dieter's plateau, which you would hit if your body knew how many calories it could expect to take in from day to day.

High-calorie days help boost your metabolic rate, maximizing the energy your body expends. Low-calorie days create a deficit, forcing your body to burn even more body fat to access the calories it needs. When you cycle from a high-calorie day to a low-calorie day, your body can't turn down its thermostat quickly enough and your metabolic rate stays high. Not only do you have a calorie deficit, but your high metabolism demands extra energy, making the deficit even bigger. You're in for maximum fat loss as you flip the fat-burning switch and make your body chase the calories!

STARTING UP

The Carb-Cycle Solution is designed to prime your body for long-term weight-loss success. You'll likely start to witness significant weight loss early on, during your first three 7-Day Carb Cycles. If you've been undereating or sumo dieting (starving in the morning and overeating late in the day), your body's been trying to survive a famine. Now you need to convince your body that it has a new, healthier lifestyle and that it's okay to lose weight. Once it learns that it will get enough calories throughout the day, your body resets its metabolism. It will finally be willing to shed those extra pounds.

Just as it takes time to break a bad habit and replace it with a good one, your body will take a little time to adjust to your new diet. This process can take a few days to a few weeks, depending on how calorie-deprived your body's been. If you've been overeating throughout the day, your body's already primed and ready to drop pounds. Every 7-Day Carb Cycle will create a beautifully balanced calorie deficit so you can start to lose weight immediately.

If after following the 7-Day Carb Cycle for three weeks you're not losing pounds or inches, be sure to read the "Troubleshooting" section at the end of this chapter. Everybody's unique, and although the weight-loss system kicks in quickly for the vast majority of people, you may need to make slight changes in the program to get results. My troubleshooting tips will answer your questions about making adjustments. Please be patient with yourself if you don't see weight loss immediately. This isn't an instant gratification diet. The Carb-Cycle Solution is a healthy way to live your life for the long term.

To start your first 7-Day Carb Cycle, begin carb cycling on the weekly schedule below. You'll notice I give you the option EITHER to take a free day once a week when you can eat anything you like (Option 1), OR to have one cheat meal of your favorite foods three days a week (Option 2). Both freebies and cheats take place on high-carb days. More on this below!

7-DAY CARB CYCLE

THE 7-DAY CARB CYCLE SCHEDULE		CHEAT MEALS / FREE DAYS
Sunday	High-Carb Day	Free Day (option 1)
Monday	Low-Carb Day	
Tuesday	High-Carb Day	Cheat Meal (option 2)
Wednesday	Low-Carb Day	
Thursday	High-Carb Day	Cheat Meal (option 2)
Friday	Low-Carb Day	
Saturday	High-Carb Day	Cheat Meal (option 2)
Saturday Morning Weigh-In		

TIMING: EAT FIVE MEALS EVERY DAY

Remember that your body is like a furnace: The hotter your metabolism gets, the more calories you burn. To stoke a furnace's fire, we feed it kindling it can burn through quickly. As the kindling burns, the furnace gets hotter, and we feed it again. And again, and again. Soon the furnace is burning so hot that we can throw in a heap of fuel, and it burns rapidly.

Your body's furnace burns every three hours. Kindling in the form of small meals eaten at those intervals keeps your metabolism burning hot. If you give it a large injection of fuel—a big meal—between the smaller meals, your body will easily burn it up.

What happens when you stop feeding the furnace? It cools down. What happens when you fuel up the furnace when it's cool? The fuel doesn't burn. It sits there, weighing down the furnace. The same thing happens when your body goes more than 3 hours without food: Your metabolic rate slows. Consume a large meal after your body's furnace cools down, and it sits there, weighing you down with fat.

Simple as that.

When you eat The Carb-Cycle Solution way, you eat at least five times every day, no matter what. It's no coincidence that almost every diet and nutrition program out there encourages you to eat smaller, frequent meals throughout the day—because it works! By eating this often, you stoke your body's metabolic furnace to incinerate anything that comes its way. What if you feel satisfied and don't feel like eating that fourth or fifth meal? Eat it anyway.

The method is easy. Eat within 30 minutes of waking, then consume a meal every 3 hours after that. Don't exceed five meals in a day. Here are examples of high-carb and low-carb schedules. The times given aren't fixed, since you might get up at a different time. It's okay if your schedule is quite different, as long as you eat every 3 hours.

Sample High-Carbohydrate Day Schedule
    6:45 am – Wake up.
    7:00 am – For breakfast, eat protein and fruit or protein and starchy carbohydrates. This turns on your metabolic furnace and fuels your body at the start of the day.
    10:00 am, 1:00 pm, 4:00 pm, and 7:00 pm – Eat protein and carbohydrates at each meal to rebuild muscle and boost your metabolism.

Sample Low-Carbohydrate Day Schedule

6:45 am – Wake up.

7:00 am – For breakfast, eat protein and fruit or protein and starchy carbohydrates. This turns on your metabolic furnace and fuels your body at the start of the day.

10:00 am, 1:00 pm, 4:00 pm, and 7:00 pm – For the remaining four meals eat protein, veggies, and fats. The combination spares muscle, regulates hormone balance, and supplies vitamins and fiber, all while BURNING FAT.

BUILDING UP TO FIVE MEALS

When you start your first 7-Day Carb Cycle, you're reprogramming your body. Remember that your body isn't used to this kind of eating pattern and it will resist the change at first. Your metabolic furnace is cold, and you need to heat it up. All your systems—digestive, nervous, muscular, endocrine, etc.—are set in their old pattern. When you start eating five meals a day, your body's going to fight against it. The first response when this happens: YOU ARE FULL. You feel stuffed, slightly uncomfortable. Three hours are going to fly by, and it's going to be time for another meal . . . and you're not going to want to eat it. But you must. Take back control with your mind! To lose weight you must eat . . . a lot.

Within about three days of starting to eat The Carb Cycle Solution way, your furnace will be heated to its maximum power for maximum weight loss. You'll no longer be full and uncomfortable, and you'll be hungry every 3 hours. Your energy levels will rise, and you'll have taken the first step to priming your body for maximum fat loss. Your body will finally begin working with you!

WHAT TO EAT FOR WEIGHT LOSS

Of course, in your five meals a day you must feed your body the right kind of food. To guide your body to a healthy weight, you need to supply it with the fuel it needs to function at its best. I've made a list of foods approved for your 7-Day Carb Cycles (see below); any food that's not on the list isn't acceptable. Certain foods that you might think of as healthy (e.g., milk and fruit juice) are missing from the list. I'll explain why.

Proteins

Protein is an absolutely critical component of weight loss. It's so important, in fact, that I require you to eat it at every meal. Protein allows your body to build muscle and prevents it from burning that muscle for energy. Muscle accounts for most of the calories you burn every day. The bigger your muscles, the more calories you burn. Muscle is your fat-burning furnace! A bonus is that your body boosts your metabolism the most when you eat protein, so eating protein causes you to burn even more calories.

Your body also uses more calories to digest protein than to digest any other food type. Although carbs crank up the metabolic thermostat, it takes more energy for your body to break down protein than any other macronutrient. You can use this to your advantage! Because it takes your body a long time (two to three hours) to fully break protein down, you'll stay fuller for longer, and you're less likely to eat more calories than you should.

Always eat your protein first, before your carbs, fats, or veggies. This way, the protein will be digested first and slow the release of other nutrients into your bloodstream. It acts like brakes on your digestion, giving you sustained energy over the next few hours.

When it comes to convenience, whey protein, which is derived from milk, is at the top of the protein list. It's an excellent immune system booster, and even people who are sensitive to cow's milk can usually handle whey with little or no problem. It comes in the form of a powder and can be found at health food stores. Choose one that's very low in fat and has less than five grams of carbohydrates per serving. A protein powder with approximately 15–20 grams of protein per serving is best. Using whey is one of the easiest ways to avoid feeling too full when eating five meals a day. Many of my clients find that drinking whey protein shakes for two or three of their five daily meals keeps them from feeling hungry or overly full. The magnificent whey protein shake is perhaps the most convenient, least expensive, most delicious protein source available.

Whey isn't the only powdered protein. For those who are severely lactose intolerant, have digestive sensitivities, or are vegan or non-lacto-vegetarian, convenient powdered proteins come from many other sources such eggs, beans, soy, rice, and hemp.

Other protein highlights:

- Cottage cheese and its low-sodium counterpart, nonfat plain Greek yogurt, contain lots of the healthy kind of bacteria, such as lactobacillus acidophilus, which aid digestion.

- Not only is fish a terrific source of protein, it often contains a significant shot of omega-3 fatty acids, the building blocks of your nervous system and brain tissue.

• For vegetarians and meat-eaters alike, soy products are an excellent source of protein. If you choose to eat soy, the fermented products, such as tempeh and tofu, are the healthiest options.

Because milk is high in both carbs and fat, it isn't included on the list of approved foods for the Carb-Cycle Solution. An average 8 ounce glass of milk, whether it's whole, reduced-fat, or skim) contains 11 or 12 grams of carbs— that's a serious hit—and whole milk can have up to 5 grams of fat. On high-carb days, you must avoid fats, and on low-carb days you can have fats but not carbs, so milk just doesn't add up for the Carb-Cycle Solution, though there are other amazing alternatives such as unsweetened almond milk.

A NOTE ABOUT DAIRY, SOY, AND WHEAT PRODUCTS

Although these can have some remarkable benefits, many people are slightly or severely intolerant of these foods—and aren't even aware of it. Sensitivities to lactose (dairy), gluten (wheat), or soy can cause inflammation in the gut and prevent nutrients from being absorbed, severely restricting your body's ability to maximize metabolic function for weight loss. Symptoms of these sensitivities are chronic gas, bloating, and gastric distress. If you have a sneaking suspicion that you may be one of the millions of Americans who are sensitive to dairy, soy, or wheat, remove the suspected culprit from your diet for two weeks, and see if you feel a difference. When you reintroduce it, your body will quickly let you know if it will tolerate the food or not!

Carbohydrates

Since you've read this far, you already know the crucial role carbohydrates play in The Carb-Cycle Solution. But all carbohydrates are not created equal, so some are noticeably missing from the list of approved foods. Carbs come in many forms, including breads, beans, potatoes, table sugar, fruits, and vegetables. Basically, if it comes from a plant, it's a carbohydrate.

There are simple carbs and complex carbs. Simple carbs are found in foods such as cakes and cookies, most commercially made bread, and many processed foods. Your body breaks down simple carbs like cane sugar and high-fructose corn syrup very quickly, spiking blood sugar levels and stimulating a massive release of insulin from the pancreas. When this happens, your blood-sugar levels rapidly drop, and you immediately begin to crave more simple carbs. Simple carbs start the vicious "crash and crave" cycle, leading to uncontrollable cravings and overeating. Because of this, simple sugary carbs aren't allowed in your 7-Day Carb Cycles, with one exception: fruit.

Although it's classified as a simple carb, fruit is loaded with vitamins, minerals, precious electrolytes, and antioxidants. But different fruits have different impacts on weight loss. Try to eat only fruit with skin on it, such as apples, peaches, apricots, grapes, nectarines, berries, and pears. The skin of these fruits is rich in fiber, which takes time to break down in your body and slows the uptake of the fruit's sugar. Like protein, fiber acts as a brake on your digestive process and the release of sugar into your bloodstream.

Fruit that you must peel before eating, such as bananas, melons, and pineapple, still have a decent amount of fiber but are not quite as weight-loss friendly. Likewise, fruit juice is low in fiber but is a highly concentrated source of sugar. I encourage you to eat fruits with skins when carb cycling, specifically in the morning. You can have your portion of fresh fruit if you eat it in your first meal of the day, and of course, you should combine it with protein such as powders, eggs, nonfat plain Greek yogurt, or cottage cheese.

Compared with simple carbs, complex carbs take much longer to digest and release into the bloodstream, so they give you a steady amount of energy over a longer period of time. In addition, complex carbs are typically high in fiber, slowing the release of sugar and digestion of food even more. Since your blood sugar remains level, and your body doesn't send hunger signals to your brain, complex carbs help curb your appetite and maximize energy output for the longest period of time. "Starches," such as true whole-grain breads and pastas (without hidden white flour or sugar), corn, peas, beans, and sweet potatoes are complex carbohydrates.

The Carb-Cycle Solution is all about complex carbs (and fruit). When I say you should have high-carb days, I mean those days should be full of complex carbs. You'll experience sustained high energy all day long!

A scale known as the glycemic index measures simple and complex carbohydrates alike. It was designed to determine how fast and how far your blood sugar rises after you eat. The foods that increase your blood sugar slowly (low glycemic index) are good, whereas foods that cause a quick rise in blood sugar (high glycemic index) aren't as desirable. Many weight-loss plans advise dieters to choose foods with low glycemic index numbers.

Although the glycemic index is a useful tool for analyzing food, The Carb-Cycle Solution doesn't rely on it for one very good reason: The system is so full of exceptions that it lacks practical application. Some of the factors that affect glycemic index include fiber content, ripeness, type of starch, fat content, acid content, physical form, cooking, processing, storage, and even how a food is cut! Who has time to figure it all out?

Let's get real: The bottom line is that you should replace highly processed grains, cereals, and sugars with minimally processed whole foods. I've selected the approved Carb-Cycle Solution carbs because they're absorbed slowly, just like low glycemic index foods (which many of them are)—no need to keep track of any numbers or the complicated glycemic index rules. Eat what's on my list, and don't worry about it!

Vegetables

Of course, vegetables are especially healthy for you. Packed with vitamins and minerals, they also contain high amounts of fiber. The health benefits of adding vegetables to your daily diet are incalculable. Vegetables nourish every system in your body, boosting your immune system, strengthening your heart, lubricating your joints, providing cancer-fighting antioxidants, and much more. Most health experts predict that you'll live longer if your diet is high in vegetables. Plus, vegetables are low in calories, making them an excellent weight-loss tool. Although technically classified as complex carbohydrates in the nutrition world, when following your 7-Day Carb Cycles you may eat life-lengthening vegetables to your heart's content and know that with every bite your body will be very grateful.

Healthy Fats

Healthy fats, namely unsaturated fats, contribute to the development and functioning of your eyes and brain and help prevent ailments such as heart disease, stroke, depression, and arthritis. The 7-Day Carb Cycles allow you to indulge in a long list of healthy fats on low-carbohydrate days, as long as you do not exceed your portion of fat per meal. Moderation is important, because healthy fats contain a lot of calorie energy and can quickly hamper your weight-loss efforts if you overindulge. It doesn't take much!

Fats are a fascinating and powerful tool for weight loss, playing a vital role in curbing your hunger. I restrict the healthy fats to low-carb days for several reasons. You're getting enough calories on high-carb days, but on low-carb days healthy fats provide some extra energy to help you feel fuller and get past the low-energy dip that you might feel. At each meal, you can have a tablespoon of natural peanut butter, a couple slices of avocado, some string cheese, or another favorite food from the fats list. These foods really help curb cravings.

Drinks

Hydrate, hydrate, hydrate! Water is imperative for loosing weight. You MUST remain hydrated throughout your journey. Ideally, you should drink eight or more TALL glasses—for a total of almost a gallon—per day. If you exercise strenuously or if the weather's hot and dry, you probably need to consume more. Some experts recommend that you drink half your body weight in ounces of water. For example, if you weigh 150 pounds, drink 75 ounces of water per day. But ideally, you should drink a gallon of water (128 ounces) every day. Use my "ten-gulp rule": Every time you take a drink, swallow ten gulps before putting the glass or bottle down. (Hint: Breathe through your nose. If ten gulps is too much, start with five and work up.) You're bound to get enough water this way!

Coffee and tea are on the approved list, but don't add sugar or milk. On low-carb days (but not on high-carb days!) you may have a tablespoon of heavy cream in your coffee, which counts as your fat portion for the meal. On both low- and high-carb days, feel free to stir in a sugar-free sweetener such as stevia or xylitol. Another great way to flavor your coffee is to blend it with a scoop of chocolate or vanilla protein powder. That way, your coffee counts as your protein for the meal!

Wean yourself off sugary sodas and energy drinks, then limit yourself to one diet soda or diet energy drink a day—only if you must. The less you drink of these chemical cocktails, the faster you'll reach your goal. I'm not a fan of the sweeteners used in most diet sodas and energy drinks, but the no-calorie options ease the transition from full-sugar drinks as you begin your weight-loss transformation. Be sure to read the labels and make certain the calorie count is low: Sugar is a big no-no, and some companies have sneaky ways of calling their drinks "diet" despite the amount of sugar they may contain.

Alcohol can greatly hinder your weight-loss efforts, so you may drink only once a week during a cheat meal. If you do choose to drink, limit yourself to beer, wine, and straight liquor. Mixed drinks are loaded with sugar and calories and can quickly destroy your weight-loss momentum. Note that alcohol is a powerful diuretic (it flushes water out of your system), so it dehydrates you, causing water retention and bloating for one to three days after you drink. Although you may not feel the effects of alcohol two days after drinking, it continues to show up in your body and on the scale. Cutting alcohol out of your diet will significantly speed up the weight-loss process.

To prevent bloating (and a hangover) after drinking alcohol, it's important to re-hydrate. Here's the secret: Before falling asleep, drink a quart of water mixed with a packet of electrolyte powder (like Emergen-C®). The electrolytes hold the water in your body like a magnet and re-hydrate you. Be sure to finish the whole quart before bedtime. When you wake in the morning, you won't have a headache, and you won't bloat for the next three days!

A FEW OUNCES OF PREVENTION

Sweeteners

Most people know that refined sugar isn't a healthy food. In fact, sugar harms your health in many ways, one being weight gain. But there's good news! You have the choice to use natural sugar substitutes that are actually good for you. Not only are stevia and xylitol beneficial to your health, they're actually just as sweet and satisfying as sugar and can easily be woven into your diet. There are plenty of other sugar substitutes, such as sucralose, aspartame, and saccharin, but I strongly suggest you go with natural sweeteners like stevia and xylitol. Both can sweeten drinks, baked goods, or anything else for that matter. You can find stevia and xylitol at your local health food store.

Stevia comes from the leaves of a bush native to the country of Paraguay. This safe alternative to sugar has been used for centuries by millions of people, notably in Japan and China. Among stevia's many health benefits are its ability to help lower blood pressure and its effectiveness as an antifungal, anti-inflammatory, and antibiotic agent. Stevia helps create balance in the pancreas, improve digestion, and reduce cavities. Many times sweeter than sugar, it can be used in small amounts. The best part about stevia is that it has almost no calories. That means you can use it whenever you want to satisfy your sweet tooth, including on low-carb days!

Xylitol is found naturally in fruits, vegetables, the bark of some trees, and even in your own body. It's been shown to reduce the bacteria that cause stomach ulcers, to eliminate sinus infections, to improve the health of the gums, sinuses, and throat, and to reduce cavities; it doesn't cause spikes in blood sugar or significantly increase your body's insulin response. Much better for your metabolism and weight-loss efforts than sugar, xylitol contains 33 percent fewer calories. Since xylitol does have more carbohydrate impact than stevia, I ask that you instead use stevia on low-carb days.

Today, more and more foods and beverages are being sweetened with stevia and xylitol, so keep an eye out for them when you want a sweet, calorie-free treat!

The Carb-Cycle Solution diet provides you with the vast majority of vitamins and minerals you need. However, I recommend you take three supplements (plus two optional ones) to help you optimize your health as you follow this program:

- A multivitamin or green-food supplement can help boost your energy on low-carb days, when you may feel sluggish. The extra energy and nutrition can also help feed your growing muscles and provide support for your body as it maintains its delicate nutrient balance.
- Probiotics help establish the healthy bacteria your colon needs to function and flourish. It's vital that you have enough healthy bacteria to digest your food, fight disease, and maintain the right nutrient balance.
- Digestive enzymes help your body break down the foods you eat. By taking enzymes before meals, you give your body that extra boost it needs to fully absorb the nutrients you feed it.
- Fish oil (optional) has been touted by both the medical and wellness communities as one of the most valuable supplements of all time. Fish oil has a multitude of benefits, from increasing "good" cholesterol and aiding brain function to supporting the production of testosterone and reducing inflammation.
- Glucosamine, chondroitin, and MSM (all optional) are the trifecta of joint-healing supplements that endurance athletes like marathoners and triathletes swear by. Your joints can certainly pay a price for the pounding they get from daily exercise. These three supplements work beautifully to reduce joint pain and inflammation.

The Approved Foods

The approved Carb-Cycle Solution grocery list isn't comprehensive—there are plenty of other good foods out there—and I invite you to visit www.chrispowell. com for more suggestions. While you're getting used to your new diet, however, it's best to eat only the foods I suggest.

If you find it difficult to taste the natural flavors of these foods at first, know that it is only temporary. The heavy sweeteners, chemicals, and additives in the unhealthy foods that you're used to have desensitized your taste buds, so they can't taste real food. Solution? Make the switch over to clean foods. After one week, your desensitized taste buds will begin to taste again. Go ahead and try some of your old foods, and you'll think you're tasting them for the first time. Sweet foods will taste even sweeter, and fatty foods will taste pretty darn greasy!

You can find information on portioning and cooking the approved foods in Chapter 15. Now stock your pantry and start eating delicious, healthy food!

THE CARB-CYCLE SOLUTION **MASTER GROCERY LIST**

PROTEIN

Dairy	Poultry	Powders	Red Meat	Seafood	Vegetable Protein
Cottage Cheese	Chicken (lean ground breast)	Egg	Buffalo (ground)	Salmon (canned in water)	Tempeh
Egg Substitutes	Chicken Breast	Legume	Beef (extra-lean ground)	Salmon (fillet)	Texturized Vegetable Protein (TVP)
Egg Whites	Chicken Thighs	Soy	Roast Beef (low-sodium deli)	Shellfish (clams, crab, lobster, mussels, scallops, shrimp)	Tofu
Yogurt (nonfat plain Greek)	Ostrich / Duck Breast	Whey	Steak (cube)		
	Turkey (breast, not deli)		Steak (cube, flank, round)	Tuna (canned in water)	
	Turkey (deli, low-sodium)		Venison /Elk	Tuna (fillet)	
	Turkey (lean ground)			White-Fleshed Fish	

CARBOHYDRATES

Bread	Breakfast Cereal	Fruit	Grain	Pasta	Root Vegetables	Starchy Vegetables	Legumes
Bread (whole-grain)	All Bran	Apples	Amaranth	Pasta (brown rice)	Potatoes (russet, red, gold; small = 1½" diameter)	Peas	Beans (boiled or low-sodium canned)
Breads (Ezekiel®)	Fiber One	Apricots	Barley	Pasta (whole-grain)		Corn	
	Granola (low-fat)	Bananas	Buckwheat				Lentils (boiled or low-sodium canned)
English Muffins (Ezekiel®)		Berries	Couscous		Sweet Potatoes / Yams (small = 2" diameter + 4" long)		
	Kashi® GOLEAN®	Grapes	Popcorn				
Tortillas (brown rice)	Kashi® Good Friends®	Kiwi	Quinoa				
	Kashi® Heart to Heart®	Melons	Rice (long-grain brown)				
Tortillas (corn)		Oranges / Tangerines					
	Oatmeal (old-fashioned or steel-cut)	Peaches / Nectarines	Rice (wild)				
Tortillas (Ezekiel®)			Spelt				
		Pears					
		Pineapple					
		Plums					

THE CARB-CYCLE SOLUTION **MASTER GROCERY LIST**

VEGETABLES

Asparagus	Carrots	Green Beans	Peppers	Turnips
Beets	Celery	Lettuce	Spinach	Zucchini
Broccoli	Collard Greens	Mixed Greens	Sprouts	
Cabbage	Cucumber	Mushrooms	Squash	
Cauliflower	Eggplant	Onions	Tomatoes	

FATS

Dairy	Dressings	Fruit	Nuts & Seeds	Oils
Cheese (low-fat)	Balsamic Vinaigrette	Avocado	Almond Butter (with salt)	Canola Oil
Egg Yolk		Olives (large)	Almonds (raw, whole)	Fish Oil
Feta Cheese	Mayonnaise (regular)		Peanut Butter (natural, with salt)	Flaxseed Oil
Heavy Cream	Salad Dressing (low-fat creamy)		Peanuts	Olive Oil
Mozzarella Cheese (low-fat)			Pecans (raw, chopped)	
			Pumpkin Seeds	
			Sesame Butter / Tahini	
			Sunflower Seeds	
			Walnuts (raw, chopped)	

DRINKS

Water	Almond Milk (unsweetened)	Coffee	Tea	

FLAVORINGS

Dressings	Herbs, Spices & Seasonings	Liquids	Tomato Products	Pastes	Sweeteners
Balsamic Vinaigrette (fat-free)	Basil	Butter Spray	Marinara Sauce	Chili Paste	Stevia
	Cayenne Pepper	Chicken Broth (low-sodium)		Hummus	Xylitol
Balsamic Vinegar	Chili Powder	Chili Sauce	Salsa	Mustard	
	Cinnamon		Tomato Paste		
Mayonnaise (fat-free / low-fat)	Cloves	Lemon Juice	Tomato Sauce		
	Cocoa Powder	Lime Juice			
Salad Dressing (fat- and sugar-free)	Curry	Soy Sauce (low-sodium)			
	Garlic				
	Ginger	Tabasco			
	Horseradish				
	Mrs. Dash® Blends				
	Nutmeg				
	Oregano				
	Parsley				
	Paprika				
	Pepper				
	Rosemary				
	Sage				
	Sea Salt				
	Tarragon				
	Thyme				
	Turmeric				

FOOD COMBINATIONS FOR MAXIMUM WEIGHT LOSS

Using the list of approved Carb-Cycle Solution foods, it's easy to get creative in the kitchen. If you're not much of a cook, the same list allows you to keep your meals as simple as you like. How you combine foods in your meals is just as important for weight loss as which foods you choose from the approved foods table. When following each 7-Day Carb Cycle, the combinations work differently on high-carb and low-carb days.

How to Eat on High-Carb Days
On high-carb days, choose at least one protein and one carbohydrate for *every* meal. If you want results fast, this is absolutely mandatory. Remember, protein is the building block that grows and maintains your muscle, and carbs are the fuel that feed your metabolic furnace. Fats, however, are off-limits on high-carb days because you're getting enough calories without them.

I always recommend you eat vegetables at every meal because they're so high in vitamins, minerals, and fiber, but they're not mandatory on high-carb days. If you're feeling quite full and you haven't eaten your vegetables yet, you don't have to eat them. I'd rather you have room for your essential macronutrients—protein and carbs. Hopefully, you can get your vegetables at your next meal. Even if you don't eat many vegetables all day, you'll probably more than make up for it tomorrow, on a low-carb day.

How to Eat on Low-Carbohydrate Days
On your low-carb days, protein is absolutely mandatory at each meal, along with vegetables and fats. The protein will help prevent your body from cannibalizing your muscle during these rapid fat-loss days, the veggies will provide vitamins, minerals, and fiber, and the fats will help curb cravings. Carbohydrates aren't an option on these days, except at breakfast. Eat a breakfast just like the high-carb day breakfast, with a combination of protein and carbs. But for the rest of the day, leave carbs out completely at every meal.

Fill up on low-carb days by choosing from the vegetables and fats lists. This is why I'm not terribly concerned if you don't eat a lot of vegetables on your high-carb days: Eating a lot of vegetables on low-carb days will make up for it. Of course, if you eat lots of vegetables every day, you'll be even healthier!

Even though you'll consume fewer calories on low-carb days, you won't go hungry. I encourage you to eat until you're satisfied. Protein and vegetables are bulky and highly nutritious, so you'll feel full before you've taken in too many calories. On low-carb days, you may feel somewhat sluggish, but embrace the feeling because it means your body's burning fat! (You're also welcome to drink some coffee or tea to give you an extra perk.) If those carb cravings come, dig in your heels, and appreciate the incredible amount of fat you're burning. You'll soon see remarkable results.

CURB THOSE CRAVINGS!

While your mind and body are making the transition to a healthier lifestyle, it's natural that you'll sometimes crave the comfort foods you used to eat. Sweets, salty snacks, and fatty foods are delicious, and it's hard to leave them behind. In each 7-Day Carb Cycle, you can still enjoy them on your free days (see the next section), but on days when you're focused on healthy eating—especially on low-carb days—it's vital that you resist temptation. The key is to manage your cravings as you experience them. Here are a few strategies that can help.

- Drink LOTS of water. It'll give you a sensation of fullness and will rein in the urge to eat when you're thirsty.

- Chew mint-flavored gum, eat a breath mint, or even put a little bit of toothpaste in your mouth . . . seriously! The mint flavor is great for suppressing your appetite and will hold you over until the next meal.

- Eat high-fiber foods early in the day. Fiber stays in your stomach and small intestine longer than low-fiber foods, keeping you full. Studies have found that people who eat high-fiber foods, such as oatmeal, in the morning are half as likely to overeat later in the day!

- Consume a little fat! Good fats, of course, and ONLY ON LOW-CARB DAYS. Simply eat one tablespoon of your favorite healthy fat, set your timer for 15 minutes, and bam! You've conquered your sweet or salty craving! Pretty cool.

FREE DAYS AND CHEAT MEALS!

Now it's time to indulge your cravings! Because let's get real: We have an emotional and psychological need for comfort foods, and it's important that they play a role in your new lifestyle. One of the most common reasons we fail on weight-loss programs is that we feel deprived. We can only hold out for so long before we give in to our cravings. The guilt and hopelessness we feel when we do can start a vicious cycle of cheating . . . and ultimately, failure.

The beautiful thing about The Carb-Cycle Solution is that you don't have to give up your favorite foods. With this plan, you're invited to take free days to enjoy the foods you crave. Yes, you can indulge in anything, from pizza to potato chips!

When it comes to the emotional and psychological release of eating the cheat foods we crave, we all work differently. Some of us prefer to stay regimented and structured for long periods of time before treating ourselves, while others prefer a more consistent reward. Because of this, I've created two cheat options.

- Option 1: Take a totally free day once a week when you can indulge in the foods you crave. It can be just one cheat meal or all of your meals for the day. Go big. Sunday is usually the best day for this. That's why we carb cyclers call it "Sunday Funday."

- Option 2: You can have a single cheat meal as often as every other day—on your high-carb days. This way, you can never fail. So how's this for a lifelong nutrition plan: If you can't have it today, you can always have it tomorrow. Sounds pretty reasonable, right?

Of course, a few rules do apply to cheat days. As long as you follow these guidelines, you can eat the pound cake *and* lose the pounds.

1. Cheat meals can only happen on high-carb days.

2. Cheat outside your house. Go to a restaurant or a convenience store, and keep the food out of the house. If it's in your house, you're going to eat it. Period. If it finds its way into your house, throw it out immediately.

3. When following Option 2, pick only one meal for your cheat meal— but it can't be dinner.

If you're one of those lucky people who don't crave junk food, all the more power to you. You'll make weight-loss progress even faster. But even if you're a junk food junkie, you'll probably start to notice that you don't crave indulgences as much as you used to. This is what happens when you fill yourself with nutritious food: Good food is quite substantial. And by eating The Carb-Cycle Solution–approved foods, you'll be cleansing your palate as well as your body. Like I said earlier, when healthy food is your main food, sweets will taste sweeter, and fatty foods will taste greasy. You may find that you lose your cravings altogether!

As you move toward greater health—and see the results of your hard work—you might want to make your cheat meals healthier by substituting better choices for your secret vices. It's far too easy to overindulge with the foods in the left-hand column below, while the healthier substitutions on the right are not just lower in calories, they help with portion control as well.

Instead of eating this:	Try this:
Candy bar or chocolate	Protein bar or chocolate protein shake
Crackers or cookies	Flavored rice cakes
Potato or tortilla chips	Popcorn
Juice or soda	Calorie-free drink
Pizza	Low-fat pizza pocket
Ice cream	Frozen yogurt or ice popsicle

MAKING YOUR MEALS EASY

Now that you know what to eat, you can make healthy high-carb and low-carb meals for yourself. I've found that the best guarantee of weight-loss success is to prepare your food ahead of time. To make the 7-Day Carb Cycle diet work for you, you must eat the right foods on the right schedule—every three hours. See Chapter 15 for examples of the wonderful meals you can enjoy on high- and low-carb days.

It's essential to make your foods in advance so that they're readily available when you need them. If you don't have the right food there for you when you're hungry, you'll go somewhere else to eat, jeopardizing your progress. Once you allow that to happen, you may allow it to happen again, and once it becomes okay the downward spiral begins.

When you prep your food in bulk, you're preparing for long-term success. For most of us, it's not practical to prepare a meal every three hours, so we have to make our food in advance. It's what I do. Like most people these days, I have an extremely busy schedule. I simply don't have the luxury of hovering over my stovetop or grill two or three times a day to make my cooked meals. So I usually cook my ingredients in bulk twice a week, on Sunday and Wednesday. Each time, I make enough to last me three or four days. Then it's simply a matter of combining the prepared ingredients and enjoying the results! I literally don't have to cook *anything* for several days, and I can still follow my diet plan.

Don't psych yourself out: Food preparation for your 7-Day Carb Cycle diet is so easy! Honestly, you can prep all your food for three or four days in about 45 minutes. That's it! By keeping your food prepped and ready to eat, you'll ensure your success on the program.

When you prepare your food in bulk, immediately portion it, and store it in separate containers. It's easiest to use plastic Tupperware®-type containers and place them in the refrigerator. Now there's no work to do for the next few days! Guaranteed success.

QUICK AND EASY ON-THE-GO FOODS

Many of my clients balk at the thought of preparing five protein-filled meals every day. It sounds like a lot, but it doesn't have to be complicated—or even cooked! I personally don't like to spend more than 5 minutes preparing a meal. If you're like me and want some quick-fix solutions that don't require any prep, these are the best foods for you:

Proteins

- Powdered proteins (whey, egg, soy, and legume powders) offer the easiest and least expensive way to get your daily protein requirements. You can substitute powdered protein for any other protein on your nutrition plan. Powders come in many different flavors, and when you mix them up, they taste like a milkshake. Another advantage is that you can quickly drink your protein and still eat your carbs or fats without feeling too full.

- Cottage cheese and nonfat, plain Greek yogurt are another great on-the-go option. You can eat them plain, combined with fruit, sweetened with stevia, or as a potato topping or sour cream substitute in recipes.

- Canned fish, chicken, and beef are other quick and convenient proteins. The quality isn't as good as fresh food, but they can be prepared as quickly as you can open the can.

- The sliced turkey, chicken, and roast beef you buy at the deli are already prepared and ready to go. Try to get the freshest cuts, preferably direct from the deli counter.

Carbohydrates

- Most fruit naturally comes in proper portion sizes. Eating fruit is a great-tasting way to rev up your metabolism first thing in the morning. Just be sure to eat your protein first or at least with the fruit.

- Low-fat/low-sugar bran cereal and granola made of high-fiber grains are perfect to portion right out of the box, especially when you're traveling.

- True whole-grain breads and tortillas (without hidden white flour or sugar) are perfect for sandwiches, wraps, and burritos, or on their own. Just toast 'em up, put 'em in the microwave or eat as is!

- Canned beans and lentils are an easily prepared source of complex carbs and protein. Open the can, heat, and enjoy. Have fun flavoring them with spices and seasonings.

- Sweet potatoes, potatoes, and yams can be cooked in the microwave with no more preparation than poking some holes in the skin or putting them in a steam bag. Each one is a perfect portion of complex carbs, ready to go.

- Oatmeal can sometimes take a little while to cook on the stovetop, but it needs just a couple minutes in the microwave. You can also use a blender to mix dry oatmeal with your protein shakes. The result is hearty and delicious and includes your protein, too. Check it out in Chapter 15!

Vegetables

- Mixed salads come already bagged in the refrigerated produce section of your grocery store.

- In just minutes, you can steam your veggies in the microwave.

- Raw veggies such as carrots, celery, cucumbers, and peppers are an incredible source of vitamins and minerals.

Fats

- Pecans, almonds, and walnuts, roasted or raw, are the healthiest choices for nuts. They're ready to eat anytime and take months to go bad. Stay away from smokehouse, salted, and other flavored nuts—they're loaded with sodium and will cause unwanted bloating.

- Avocadoes are a great source of healthy fats, and they go great with protein and veggies alike.

- Salad dressing adds flavor to vegetables without mess or fuss. Vinaigrettes are usually the healthiest choice; you may also have low-fat creamy dressings like blue cheese and ranch in moderation according to your portions, but avoid sweet, sugary dressings completely. Note that there can be a lot of hidden sodium in salad dressing, which can cause bloating. Use it in moderation, and stick with your approved portions!

- Low-fat cheese supplies wonderful, healthy fat. String or sliced cheese is easily portioned for your meal plan.

- Peanut butter (the natural kind) is one of my favorites—I know I'm not alone here! One tablespoon goes a LONG way on its own or as flavoring in a meal.

TRACKING YOUR SUCCESS

Along the road to any destination, signs tell us where we are and how far we have to go. On the transformation highway, you can get a lot of encouragement by reading the signs of your progress. One sign, your weight, takes the longest to change, so it's the last one you should look to when judging your transformation. Several other signs can tell you where you are on your way to success.

READ THE **ROAD SIGNS**

	HIGH-CARB DAY	**LOW-CARB DAY**
Energy	High	Low
Thinking	Clear	Slow
Water	Retention	Flush
Body Temp	High	Low
Cravings	Low	Moderate
Weight	Stable or slight rise	Drop
Muscle Endurance	Increased AFTERWARD	Decreased AFTERWARD

Sign #1: Clothing and Inches
Pay attention to how your clothes fit. This is the BEST gauge of your progress. Periodically taking your body measurements can also be useful.

Sign #2: Energy Levels, Mental Clarity, and Body Temperature
As your body burns through lots of readily available calories on high-carb days, you'll notice a nice boost of energy and a rise in your body temperature. At night, you may even find yourself stripping the blankets off the bed because you're so hot. Low-carb days come with decreased energy levels and body temperature. Don't be alarmed if you feel a bit lethargic and foggy-minded without all those carbs, especially at first. This is normal, and it's only temporary, until you switch back to a high-carb day. If you're having high- and low-energy swings from one

day to the next, you're right on track! Pay attention to this because your body will guide the way.

If you find you're sluggish on low-carb days and need a pick-me-up, green tea is an excellent boost for mental clarity and energy. I'm not opposed to a cup of coffee here and there, either. You'll find that your sensitivity to caffeine will increase significantly, so enjoy a small or medium cup, and avoid the extra-large triple-shot café Americano!

Sign #3: Appetite and Cravings

Low-carb days typically bring increased appetite and cravings. Oh boy . . . sweet potatoes are ten times more appetizing on my low-carb days! Conversely, as you load your body with energy on high-carb days, you'll notice that your appetite and cravings are minimal. When you experience cravings (especially for carbs), one of the best tricks of the trade is to curb those cravings …with a glass of water, mint flavored gum, or a breath mint. If you're craving a cookie, have a tablespoon of natural peanut butter, a stick of string cheese, a few slices of avocado, or a portion of any of the other acceptable fats on the list instead. Within 15 minutes of eating healthy fat, your appetite will be satisfied, and you won't want the foods you craved. Easy!

If you retain a lot of water on a regular basis, check your sodium intake. You might be retaining water because you're getting too much sodium in your diet. Water retention from excess sodium intake can increase your weight by 5–15 pounds!

The United States has one of the highest-sodium diets in the world because of the enormous amounts of sodium hidden in our food. Assuming you've cut processed foods out of your diet, meats and flavorings are the two main sodium culprits. Search for fresh meats that aren't "plumped" (injected with sodium). Most deli meats are incredibly high in sodium, but there are low-sodium turkey and roast beef options. Often, sauces and flavorings (even some of those on the acceptable foods list), from mustard to soy sauce, are incredibly high in sodium. Read your labels, and use your sauces and flavorings sparingly for accurate weigh-ins.

If you reduce your sodium intake to less than the suggested daily maximum of 2,400 mg (or ideally, to the recommended 1,500 mg), your body will stop bloating from excess water over the course of three days.

POUR OFF SOME **POUNDS**

91

Sign #4: Water Retention and Flushing

It's one more reason NOT to rely only on the scale: Your body will naturally retain water on high-carb days and will flush it on low-carb days. Your weight will fluctuate as a result. When you eat carbs and drink water, the water sticks to you like Velcro®. No need to worry about this. You'll flush the water on the following low-carb day. What do I mean by flush? Basically, you're going to urinate a lot, sometimes even a couple times every hour! Whatever you do, don't scale back on your water. Stay hydrated and appreciate your body's response to carb cycling. This is a beautiful sign!

Sign #5: Sleep

Carbohydrates often prompt your brain to release a hormone called serotonin, which helps you relax and aids in sleep. Since you won't be taking in carbohydrates on your low-carb days, you may find it more difficult to fall asleep for the first few nights following those days. Meditate, breathe deeply, take a warm bath, or read something relaxing to help you fall asleep. Many people have no problem at all, but if you're one of the sensitive few, remember that your body will adapt. Hang in there.

Sign #6: Weight

It's logical that people seeking to lose weight typically try to gauge their success by weighing themselves. A scale can definitely be your friend when measuring weight loss, but weighing yourself daily won't give you a true or accurate picture of your progress. Your weight fluctuates on a day-to-day basis when you're going through the 7-Day Carb Cycle, so weighing yourself is valuable only once a week. Make Saturday your weekly weigh-in day, and watch the pounds drop away. If you just *have to* weigh yourself daily, you'll notice an increase in your weight after high-carb days and a decrease after low-carb days. This is natural and expected, so if you see these fluctuations, you know you're on track!

Keep in mind that it will be roughly one to two weeks before you get a truly meaningful reading on the scale. For the first several weeks of the program, you may actually maintain your starting weight but lose inches and clothing sizes. This may be due to *recomposition*, when your body starts building muscle, burning fat, and shedding water all at the same time. Recomposition takes only a couple of weeks while your body adjusts to your new diet and exercise routine. Soon you'll notice a drop on the scale as muscle-gain slows and fat-burning increases.

TROUBLESHOOTING

If you've been following the 7-Day Carb Cycles for a few weeks and have either remained at your starting weight or noticed no difference in the way your clothes fit, it's time to take a step back and tweak your program to get your weight-loss going. The same goes if you're within ten pounds of your ideal weight and your weight-loss has slowed or stopped. Ask yourself these questions:

Am I Eating Five Meals a Day?
Whenever my clients tell me, "I'm following the program and I'm not noticing any differences," I reply, "How many meals are you eating each day?" Almost without fail they say, "It's just so hard to eat all that food. I'm getting maybe three meals." Well, my friend, if you're one of these people, then we've already nailed down your problem. You *must* eat five meals every day. Your body needs to know that it doesn't have to store calories, that more food is just around the corner. Its evolutionary habit of gaining fat to use in case of a failed hunt or a poor harvest no longer works. When you strictly follow the 7-Day Carb Cycle, your body learns it's okay to burn fat. You must consistently feed your body approved foods every three hours, five times a day. Most people who follow this protocol will lose weight.

Am I Getting Too Many Calories?
First, troubleshoot your cheat meals. Do you find yourself unable to control yourself during cheat meals? Of course, you're allowed to indulge in your favorite foods during a cheat meal in moderation, but if these foods are triggers and the indulgences turn into bingeing, avoiding those foods may be the best option for now. You may want to consider reducing your cheat meals to just one free day per week.

Remember, cheat meals are designed to reward you psychologically and emotionally, not to become an excuse to binge. If you do need some kind of regular daily food reward, look to calorie-free solutions such as flavored waters to satisfy any sweet cravings.

Next, analyze your daily food intake. Eating too much, of course, makes weight loss impossible. Misjudging your portion sizes can make a big difference in your progress. Stick to the fast and easy hand portion guidelines I've given for portioning your foods (See Chapter 15). If you still experience no change on the scale after a few weeks, you may want to try reducing your portions by about one-quarter from what you are currently eating to see how your body reacts.

If you are ever in doubt about portion size, use the 100-calorie chart of all acceptable foods to add up your calories. Using hand portions is practical and easy, but adding up your calories will let you know exactly what the issue may be.

Keep in mind that the amount of calories on high- and low-carb days should be different! For the most dramatic results, an average woman may consume 1,200 calories on a low-carb day and 1,500 calories on a high-carb day. An average man may consume 1,500 calories on a low-carb day and 2,000 calories on a high-carb day.

Am I Not Eating Enough Calories?

If you are ever in doubt, use the 100-calorie chart of all the acceptable foods to make sure that you are actually eating enough. I know it is a pain to measure your foods, but when you're trying to lose weight, it is SO important to use those measuring cups and verify that your portions are as recommended for your 7-Day Carb Cycling.

Keep in mind that women should never eat less than 1,200 calories a day, and men should never eat less than 1,500 calories. As explained earlier in this book, your body has built-in survival mechanisms that slow your metabolism when your calorie intake gets dangerously low. To make sure you are getting enough calories, use the 100-calorie portion charts to find out exactly how many calories you are consuming on your high- and low-carb days.

Am I Getting My Daily Exercise?

If so, fantastic. You're on your way to a lean and fit body. It's important to understand that when you begin resistance (weight) training, you'll most likely gain muscle. Don't worry—normal humans don't have the hormonal capacity to grow to the size of most bodybuilders! You'll naturally grow a little bit of muscle, and then you'll stop. However, keep in mind that muscle weight will show up on the scale, so don't freak out if you see your numbers stay the same or rise a pound or two, even if you start dropping clothing sizes like crazy! Your body is going through recomposition, gaining muscle and losing fat. This is a good thing. Let your body grow the muscle until it's done, then watch the pounds drop off.

But I'm Really, Truly Following The Program!

What if you're in the small percentage who strictly follow the program and still don't see results? You'll need to make adjustments in order to make it work for you. Although our bodies all go by the same weight-loss principles, the point at which the 7-Day Carb Cycle kicks in can be slightly different for each of us. All it should take to get you on track is a minor tweak on your high-carb days:

- Include carbs and protein in your first three meals of the day.

- Remove carbs from your last two meals.

- Eat protein, vegetables, and fat for your last two meals.

This should kick-start your weight loss!

THE 7-DAY CARB CYCLE GUIDELINES

- Eat high-carb and low-carb meals on alternate days.

- Eat five meals every day.

- Choose from the list of approved foods.

- Measure the right portion sizes for YOU.

- On low-carb days, eat a high-carb breakfast that combines one portion of protein and one portion of carbs. Cut carbs completely from the rest of your meals, and include one portion each of protein and fats. Eat as many vegetables as you can.

- On high-carb days, at all five of your daily meals, include one portion of carbs and one portion of protein; vegetables are highly recommended.

- Eat within 30 minutes of waking and every 3 hours thereafter.

- Drink a gallon of water daily.

CHAPTER 10:
QUICK-START GUIDE

Like many of my clients, you might want to get a running start on The Carb-Cycle Solution. Here it is in a nutshell. Refer to the chapters indicated for details. Get ready for a great 7-Day Carb Cycle!

1. FUEL UP

Set the stage for proper nutrition by stocking up and prepping a week's worth of ingredients:

- Buy a week's worth of the foods you like from the "Approved Foods" section of Chapter 9.

- Find your portions based on your current weight. See the Master Portion List in Chapter 15.

- Select from the recipes provided in Chapter 15, or create your own meals based on your proper portions. Prepare a week's worth of ingredients for the recipes you have chosen. You should make enough food for five meals a day on each of your four high-carb days and three low-carb days.

CARB INTAKE	NUMBER OF DAYS PER WEEK	DAILY NUMBER/TYPE OF MEALS
High-Carb Days	4 days	5 high-carb meals
Low-Carb Days	3 days	1 high-carb breakfast PLUS 4 low-carb meals

CARB **DAYS**

97

2. FOLLOW THE 7-DAY CARB CYCLE SCHEDULE

Eat a high-carb diet on one day and a low-carb diet on the next, alternating throughout the week. If you like, take a day off on Sunday to eat whatever you want.

WEEKLY **DIET**

DAY OF THE WEEK	DAILY DIET
Sunday	High-Carb/FREE Day
Monday	Low-Carb Day
Tuesday	High-Carb Day
Wednesday	Low-Carb Day
Thursday	High-Carb Day
Friday	Low-Carb Day
Saturday	High-Carb Day/Morning Weigh-In

• Eat within 30 minutes of waking and every 3 hours afterward, for five meals a day.

3. CHOOSE YOUR REWARD

The 7-Day Carb Cycle builds in opportunities for you to indulge in your favorite foods. You can schedule your splurges in one of two ways:

- • Option 1: Eat according to the 7-Day Carb Cycle schedule, and take a full free day on Sunday. Eat anything you want, all day long. This option tends to yield the best results. OR

- • Option 2: Eat one cheat meal on each high-carb day. Your cheat meal cannot be dinner.

3. DRINK A GALLON OF WATER EVERY DAY

That's 128 ounces, a little more than ten 12-ounce glasses a day.

4. DO YOUR SHAPERS

Complete a ten-minute shaper workout first thing in the morning every other day on your low-carb days. The "Shapers" section of Chapter 12 tells you everything you need to know about these resistance/weight-training exercises.

Monday	• Low-Carb Day	• Sprint Shaper Circuits
Wednesday	• Low-Carb Day	• Endurance Shaper Circuits
Friday	• Low-Carb Day	• Shape & Size Shaper Circuits

5. DO YOUR SHREDDERS

Every day, six days a week, do a five-shredder, 30-minute workout. If you aren't used to exercise, you can do two shredders (12 minutes) a day and work up to five. The "Shredders" section of Chapter 12 tells you everything you need to know about these fat-burning cardio intervals.

6. WEIGH IN ON SATURDAY

Especially during your first 7-Day Carb Cycle, don't step on the scale every day. You'll see too many fluctuations and the numbers will be meaningless. Instead, weigh yourself only once, before breakfast on Saturday morning.

7. RELAX ON SUNDAY

Don't do any shapers or shredders on your rest day: Your body needs time to rest and recover from exercise. Sunday is your free day—eat anything you want! If you choose to stick with The Carb-Cycle Solution–approved foods, make this a high-carb day. Now you're on your way. Go for it!

CHAPTER 11:
THE SLINGSHOT TECHNIQUE

Carbohydrate cycling isn't the end of the weight-loss process. Some people react quickly to the 7-Day Carb Cycle and can keep losing for a long time. Others lose at first but then quickly plateau. No matter what pattern your body follows, it WILL eventually begin to adapt to carb cycling and stop losing weight. Carb cycling is probably the most effective way to offset your body's ability to adapt to weight loss, but as with every diet plan, your weight loss will probably plateau eventually.

If your weight loss stalls or stops, it means that your highly intelligent body has learned the 7-Day Carb Cycle pattern and is adapting to conserve as much energy (fat) as possible. In other words, you've hit the dreaded dieter's plateau. When carb cycling, your body may reach this stage anytime between the second and twelfth weeks. But you don't have to quit and just accept whatever weight loss you've already achieved. In fact, this is when The Carb-Cycle Solution really gets fun! At this point, when your amazing body starts to decipher the code, you once again turn the tables with the slingshot technique.

The slingshot technique is absolutely critical to sustaining weight loss because during this week, your body is convinced to reset and boost your metabolism. A body with a high metabolism is a body that knows it can count on getting lots of healthy food, so it freely converts calories into energy rather than storing them as fat.

WHAT IS THE SLINGSHOT TECHNIQUE?

On other weight-loss programs, the dieter's plateau would be a frustrating problem. But on The Carb-Cycle Solution, it's easily resolved. Even better, the antidote is built into the program. Your body has figured out your 7-Day Carb Cycle pattern and stopped losing weight. Change your eating pattern when this happens, and your body has to work to adapt again. This restarts your metabolism, so you can break through your weight-loss wall and lose even more.

By using the slingshot technique, you won't get stuck on the dieter's plateau—you'll race right across it and down the other side! All you need to do is to "periodize" your weekly nutrition, which is what the slingshot technique allows you to do. Periodization is the practice of constantly changing the way you eat. It's the single most effective way to keep your body from figuring out what you're trying to do!

To slingshot, take seven high-carbohydrate days in a row. This revs your metabolism, fills your body with nutritious food, and absolutely primes you to lose weight again. Your body will notice you're not having any low-calorie (low-carb) days, and it will assume there's no reason to conserve. You'll start burning tons of calories. That's your metabolic boost. Once your metabolism pumps up on carbs in your slingshot week, you throw it a curveball by dropping back into a 7-Day Carb Cycle the very next week.

No matter how adaptive your system, it can't adjust in time, and weight loss is inevitable. Basically, with the slingshot technique you clear the slate to restart your weight loss. Simply alternate between three 7-Day Carb Cycles and one week of slingshotting until you've reached your desired weight. So there you have it—the secret to consistent and permanent weight loss. No more mystery to the dieter's plateau. Now YOU are in control!

HOW TO WORK THE SLINGSHOT TECHNIQUE

At some point on their journey to transformation, my clients inevitably say, "My weight loss has slowed down." To that I usually respond, "Eat more!" When they increase their food consumption, their weight loss actually picks up speed. You won't gain weight, even though you're eating a lot more. Your intuitive response to a dieter's plateau will probably be to eat less and exercise more. DON'T DO IT! You'll just get more firmly stuck where you are. What you need is a slingshot!

So how do you implement the slingshot technique and guarantee that your body will keep losing weight? It's unbelievably simple. After following the 7-Day Carb Cycle for three weeks, take one slingshot week to rev up your metabolic engine.

Depending on your body, your weight may remain the same during this week, or you may lose a significant amount of weight. Any slight weight gain you may see is due solely to water retention, and the water will flush as you return to your 7-Day Carb Cycles. If you level off instead of losing, don't worry.

When you resume 7-Day Carb Cycling, you'll be past the plateau and will start losing weight again.

So don't vary the protocol. Stay on course!

Guidelines for the Slingshot Technique:

- For one week, every day is a high-carb day.
- Eat five meals every day.
- Choose from the list of approved foods.
- Measure the right portion sizes for YOU.
- At all five of your daily meals, include one portion of carbs and one portion of protein; vegetables are highly recommended.
- Eat within 30 minutes of waking and every three hours thereafter.
- Drink a gallon of water daily.

YIKES! IT'S NOT WORKING!

Many people only need to alternate three 7-Day Carb Cycles with one-week of the slingshot technique to reach their ideal weight. However, the impact of the carb-cycle/slingshot pattern varies quite a bit from person to person. Your body may require a greater adjustment period to reset its metabolism and gear itself up for continued weight loss. If you don't lose weight after you slingshot, you'll need to tweak the program a bit to get the results you want. The "Troubleshooting" section at the end of Chapter 9 offers alternative carb cycling options for people with stubborn bodies.

CHAPTER 12:
GET MOVING

"To have a functioning body and not to use it is like having
20/20 vision and never opening your eyes."
—Bill Phillips, fitness pioneer and author of *Body for Life*

Your body is a machine that's built to move. Your legs are made to run, walk, skip, dance, and jump. Your arms and hands are made to push, pull, wave, hug, and hold. Your spine can flex and extend to bend and reach. When it does what it was designed to do—MOVE—your body is healthiest and happiest. Your muscles want to be used. Do your body a favor and make it move every day!

Exercise benefits your body in numerous ways, and scientists are discovering more positive effects with each new study. People who make exercise a priority have lower rates of cancer, heart disease, and high blood pressure. More oxygen is available to every organ of their body, and their muscles are stronger. Regular exercisers have lower rates of depression and other mental disorders. They have more energy and feel better than non-exercisers. And yes, people who exercise are much more likely to have lean, muscular, sexy bodies. Exercise is a vital factor in losing weight and keeping it off forever.

Can you follow The Carb-Cycle Solution and lose weight without exercising? Sure. Nutrition is the most powerful driving force behind weight loss, accounting for the majority of your weight-loss success. But if you write off exercise, you won't reach your full health potential. Carbohydrate cycling will definitely change your body composition, but your rate of weight loss and your overall strength and endurance will be incomparably greater if you also exercise. It's critical for every human body to be put into motion if it is to achieve optimal health.

With all the hard work you're putting into losing weight, you surely don't want your triumph to be temporary! You want to lose that weight forever. By integrating exercise into your life, you make a commitment to *permanent* weight loss.

THE ULTIMATE WORKOUT PROGRAM FOR *YOU*

As a fitness student and professional with many years of experience, I know literally hundreds of exercises that I could have incorporated into an exercise program geared to weight loss. The system I've designed for The Carb-Cycle Solution is the product of extensive practice, painstaking study, and careful fine-tuning. It's the most effective and time-efficient workout possible, and it deliberately amplifies the effects of carb cycling. The workouts will help you gain muscle, endurance, and a high level of fitness so you can reach your weight-loss goals in half the time of dieting alone, and yet you will be blown away by how simple they are.

Most exercise experts divide workouts into two categories: cardiovascular (aerobic) exercise and resistance (anaerobic) exercise. Cardiovascular exercises like walking, jogging, and bicycle riding are typically sustained, lower-intensity movement for a prolonged period—amazing for burning calories, but they can't significantly improve the size, shape, or strength of your muscles. In fact, during cardiovascular exercise your body tries to burn muscle as you lose fat, so you need regular resistance training to build and maintain your precious muscle—the main component of your metabolic furnace. The fastest way to lose fat is to keep your metabolic furnace burning as hot as possible: If you keep stimulating your muscles, you'll reach your weight-loss goal SO much faster than by relying on nutrition and cardio alone.

I call The Carb-Cycle Solution's resistance-training circuits *shapers* because they boost your metabolism by building and shaping your muscle. The Carb-Cycle Solution cardiovascular intervals, which I call *shredders*, burn fat like crazy. The more you shred, the more body fat you burn. Shapers and shredders accomplish different goals, so combining them into a complete fitness plan is the best way to achieve weight loss and overall health. The Carb-Cycle Solution program devotes three days a week to a 10-minute resistance shaper workout, and you do your 6-minute shredders six days a week. The remaining day of the week is for rest.

I've designed short workouts to make it super-easy to fit the exercise program into your schedule. Another great thing about them is that you don't have to join a gym or buy expensive equipment to follow the program. You can do the shapers on your living room floor, and you can get most of your shredders done outdoors. Your body is the only equipment you need, because you can do every exercise by using your own body weight. In fact, that's what we're built for—mastering our own body weight!

Best of all, you don't need to spend a lot of time and money exercising to accomplish fantastic results. I'll show you exactly how to use your time so that every minute of your exercise session counts.

GETTING STARTED

If you're not accustomed to exercising regularly, I urge you to *ease* into this program. The workout is designed to be challenging, and most people aren't immediately comfortable with all the exercises. For now, just by putting your body into motion you'll begin to reap wonderful results. Take it slowly, focus on what you can do, and make it a goal to improve with each workout. If at any time you feel light-headed or short of breath, sit down and relax. Your workouts should be intense but enjoyable, so give yourself permission to increase the intensity and length of each session gradually. If you're consistent, you will notice results, even if you take it easy at first. Before long, you'll be amazed at your performance.

As your workouts become part of your new and healthier lifestyle, you'll likely begin to look forward to this special time in your day. This is when you're doing something for yourself—investing in your health and your future. Your workouts are among the most important daily commitments that you make to yourself. They're an opportunity to grow your integrity—the value you place on yourself—every day. Working out will make you feel better physically, mentally, and emotionally. Most people who incorporate regular exercise into their life can't imagine going back to their old couch-potato lifestyle. Once you join the millions of active daily exercisers, I'm confident you'll never look back.

You should jump right into your morning shaper as soon as you wake up on your low-carb days. It'll get your metabolism going and put your body into high gear for the day. Do your shredders anytime after that—immediately following your shapers or in the late morning, early afternoon, or even the evening. Whenever works best for you!

The long-lasting effects of morning exercise are astounding. If you start the day with a workout—even just a quick 10-minute session—you'll notice increased energy and productivity throughout the day. You'll also find that you sleep more soundly at night when you work out in the morning.

Even better, you'll probably need less sleep, since your sleep will be deeper. That makes it easier to set your alarm earlier to get your morning exercise. It may be difficult to wake up at first, but after three to five days, your body alarm will automatically get you up in time for your morning shaper!

WORKOUT WAKE-UP

BEFORE AND AFTER YOUR WORKOUT

Whether you're doing shapers, shredders, or both, always remember to warm up before your workouts, and cool down when you're done. It's unwise to shock your body by starting exercise without a warm-up to prevent injury. Another bad idea is to stop exercising without giving your body a chance to cool down. Cooling down keeps your blood from pooling in your extremities and lets your heart and lungs gear down slowly.

A great warm-up for these workouts is to march in place for one minute, then jog in place for 30 seconds, and finally do jumping jacks for the last 30 seconds. These exercises move some of the biggest muscle groups in your body and help increase your body temperature and blood flow to your muscles and joints. If you warm up, your muscles will be able to contract and relax faster. Plus, you'll be less likely to suffer strains and pulls. Ultimately, 5 minutes is ideal for a warm-up, but let's get real: You've got a busy life and need to get going. If you warm up for at least 2 minutes, you'll do your body a world of good. Your body's warm when you begin to break a light sweat.

Before Your Workout

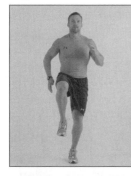 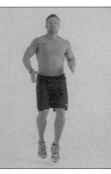 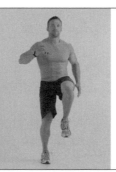

Marching
1 minute

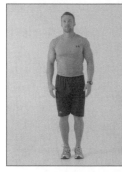 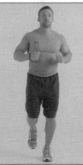 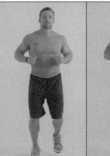 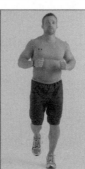

Jogging in Place
30 seconds

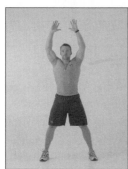 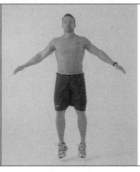

Jumping Jacks
30 seconds

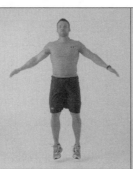 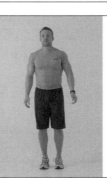

Jumping Jacks

109

For your cool-down, simply finish with 3 minutes of light-intensity cardio, such as walking.

That's it! Now you're ready to rock your workout!

SHAPERS

Muscle-building exercise uses body-weight resistance to boost your metabolic rate. I call resistance-exercise circuits *shapers*, a term meant to help you remember why you do them. Shapers are key to developing the shape and strength of your muscles, an important part of your weight-loss plan because the bigger your muscles, the higher your metabolism. When your metabolism is high, weight loss is much easier to accomplish. Plus, bigger muscles require more calories around the clock.

Each muscle group need only resist a strong force—a heavy weight or an immovable object such as a wall or floor—for a few minutes every other day to receive the stimulus it needs to grow. The improved shape of your muscles comes from an increase in the size of individual muscle fibers as well as an increase in the number of muscle cells.

Always do your shapers after high-carb days, when your muscles are fueled up and ready for maximum performance. On The Carb-Cycle Solution, you'll do your shapers on Monday, Wednesday, and Friday, your low-carb days. (If your schedule doesn't allow this, you can always do them on Tuesday, Thursday, and Saturday, and make those your low-carb days.) The best way to maximize your weight loss is to wake up in the morning and do your shapers, and then eat breakfast.

Following your morning shaper workout, eat a high-protein and high-carbohydrate breakfast (which replenishes carbs burned during the workout and reduces cortisol), then cut out carbs for the rest of the day. By aligning carbohydrate cycling with shapers, you set the stage for the fastest weight loss.

DON'T RUSH IT!

The first few times you do your shapers, try to go with the flow and get a feel for the exercises. You should allow more time for your first few sessions, so you can get used to the movements. If they seem awkward at first, hang in there! Once you're familiar with the shaper workout, it will only take you 10 minutes in the morning.

No matter your fitness level, start the program slowly and carefully until you are both mentally comfortable with and physically capable of performing the moves correctly. Just like when you learn to ride a bike, your body needs to get used to the movements before you can smooth them out.

Don't push it. So many people approach their workouts with a "no pain, no gain" mentality, which only leads to overtraining and failure—and sometimes injury. Your success and safety is paramount, so don't exercise any faster or harder than feels right. Be patient with yourself if you get winded. With time and practice, the movements will get easier.

In just a little while, you'll get into the groove. When you feel comfortable enough, try closing your eyes during each exercise and focusing on the contraction of individual muscles. This will help you gain an understanding of your body in motion.

GETTING FITTER FASTER

It is simple: The term is Progressive Overload, and it is the underlying principle behind you getting fitter, faster. Each and every week aim to perform either more reps or more rounds than you did in the last workout of the same type. Within the first few weeks you will notice an incredible jump in the amount of reps and rounds you can perform in each workout. At times you may plateau for a couple of weeks, but keep striving and challenging yourself for more. As long as you continue to improve in the number of repetitions and rounds that you are capable of performing in each of the three workouts, you will continue to see and feel an incredible difference in your body. You will be getting fitter!

THE SHAPER CIRCUITS

After years of research into thousands of possible shaper exercises, I shaved The Carb-Cycle Solution workout down to the only three you'll ever need to know: the push-up, the sit-up, and the squat. These three exercises cover the fundamental movements of your body: pushing, crunching, and squatting. (Using body weight alone, it's difficult to incorporate pulling motions, so those aren't included.) When brought together, push-ups, sit-ups, and squats work nearly all your muscles. You'll be very surprised at what an incredible workout you can get using just these three movements!

Shapers mirror the motions you make in everyday life. The workout includes squats to help you get up and down out of cars and chairs, sit-ups to help you engage your core muscles, and push-ups for getting up off the ground and pushing away from objects. In only 10 minutes a day you'll gain greater strength, muscle endurance, and stamina for everyday activities—not to mention lose a lot of weight. As you become more conditioned, you'll be able to do more and more circuits. Each week, challenge yourself to perform more rounds and more repetitions than the last. This is the only way your fitness improves!

There are 3 different types of shaper workouts:

Sprint

1. Perform three sit-ups, six push-ups, and nine squats to complete one circuit.

2. Do as many circuits as you can in 10 minutes. Fast-moving and high-intensity, this kind of sprint circuit has been shown to trigger a significant increase in metabolic rate for many hours post-exercise, meaning that your body will be a fat-burning furnace throughout your morning!

Endurance

1. Perform as many sit-ups as you can in 20 seconds. Rest for ten seconds.

2. Again, do as many repetitions as you can in 20 seconds. Rest for ten seconds.

3. Continue for six rounds, for a total of three minutes.

4. Repeat the process for push-ups and squats. These circuits stimulate your muscle for endurance and stamina. During the movements, a significant burn will build up in your muscle. This is completely natural and expected! As you incinerate the carbohydrates in your muscle, lactic acid builds up, and you feel the burn. Your muscle will demand more calories to keep moving, and it will find what it needs in your fat. For the rest of your low-carb day, your body is forced to burn even more fat for fuel.

Shape & Size
1. Perform 10 squats and 10 push-ups. This equals one round.
2. Do as many of these rounds as you can in five minutes.
3. Perform 10 squats and 10 sit-ups. This equals one round.
4. Do as many rounds as you can in five minutes.

YOUR SHAPER SCHEDULE

Sunday	Rest
Monday	Sprint Shaper
Tuesday	Rest
Wednesday	Endurance Shaper
Thursday	Rest
Friday	Shape & Size Shaper
Saturday	Rest

SAMPLE SHAPER TRAINING PROGRESSION

Beginner	Week 1	Week 2	Week 3	Week 4	Week 5	Week 6
Sprint Circuit total rounds:	5 rounds	5 rounds	6 rounds	6 rounds	6 rounds	7 rounds
Endurance Circuit reps per each exercise:	30 reps	32 reps	34 reps	36 reps	38 reps	40 reps
Shape & Size Circuit 1	3 rounds	3 rounds	3 rounds	4 rounds	4 rounds	4 rounds
Circuit 2	3 rounds	3 rounds	4 rounds	3 rounds	3 rounds	4 rounds
Intermediate	**Week 1**	**Week 2**	**Week 3**	**Week 4**	**Week 5**	**Week 6**
Sprint Circuit total rounds:	10 rounds	10 rounds	10 rounds	11 rounds	11 rounds	11 rounds
Endurance Circuit reps per each exercise:	50 reps	52 reps	54 reps	56 reps	58 reps	60 reps
Shape & Size Circuit 1	6 rounds	6 rounds	6 rounds	6 rounds	7 rounds	7 rounds
Circuit 2	4 rounds	4 rounds	4 rounds	5 rounds	5 rounds	5 rounds
Advanced	**Week 1**	**Week 2**	**Week 3**	**Week 4**	**Week 5**	**Week 6**
Sprint Circuit total rounds:	15 rounds	15 rounds	15 rounds	16 rounds	16 rounds	17 rounds
Endurance Circuit reps per each exercise:	70 reps	72 reps	74 reps	76 reps	78 reps	80 reps
Shape & Size Circuit 1	8 rounds	8 rounds	8 rounds	8 rounds	9 rounds	9 rounds
Circuit 2	5 rounds	5 rounds	6 rounds	6 rounds	6 rounds	6 rounds

Beginner	Week 7	Week 8	Week 9	Week 10	Week 11	Week 12
Sprint Circuit total rounds:	7 rounds	7 rounds	8 rounds	8 rounds	9 rounds	9 rounds
Endurance Circuit reps per each exercise:	42 reps	44 reps	46 reps	48 reps	50 reps	52 reps
Shape & Size Circuit 1	4 rounds	5 rounds	5 rounds	5 rounds	5 rounds	5 rounds
Circuit 2	4 rounds	4 rounds	5 rounds	4 rounds	4 rounds	5 rounds
Intermediate	**Week 7**	**Week 8**	**Week 9**	**Week 10**	**Week 11**	**Week 12**
Sprint Circuit total rounds:	12 rounds	12 rounds	13 rounds	13 rounds	14 rounds	14 rounds
Endurance Circuit reps per each exercise:	62 reps	64 reps	66 reps	68 reps	70 reps	72 reps
Shape & Size Circuit 1	7 rounds	7 rounds	7 rounds	8 rounds	8 rounds	8 rounds
Circuit 2	5 rounds	6 rounds	6 rounds	5 rounds	6 rounds	6 roudns
Advanced	**Week 7**	**Week 8**	**Week 9**	**Week 10**	**Week 11**	**Week 12**
Sprint Circuit total rounds:	17 rounds	18 rounds	18 rounds	19 rounds	19 rounds	19 rounds
Endurance Circuit reps per each exercise:	82 reps	84 reps	86 reps	88 reps	90 reps	92 reps
Shape & Size Circuit 1	9 rounds	9 rounds	10 rounds	10 rounds	10 rounds	10 rounds
Circuit 2	7 rounds	7 rounds	7 rounds	8 rounds	8 rounds	8 rounds

THE SHAPER EXERCISES

As you can see, there are only three shaper exercises: sit-ups, push-ups, and squats. Depending on your fitness level, you can do each of these exercises at three different intensities, from beginner to intermediate to advanced. Each week, challenge yourself to perform more repetitions than the last. This is the only way your fitness will improve. It's time to get to the meat of the matter!

Sit-Ups
Beginner Sit-Ups (knee pops)

1 Lie flat on the floor with arms overhead, knees bent at a 90-degree angle, and feet tucked under a sofa or heavy armchair.

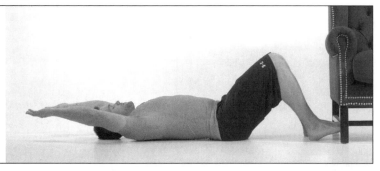

2 Swing arms forward and sit up, crunching forcefully with your abdominal muscles.

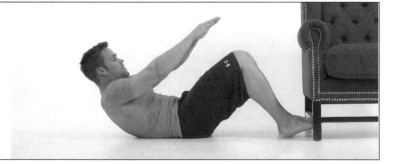

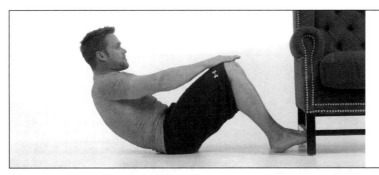

3 Slap the top of your knees with your palms to mark the top of the rep.

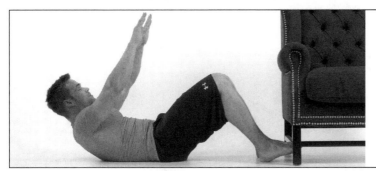

4 Return to the lying-down position to complete the rep.

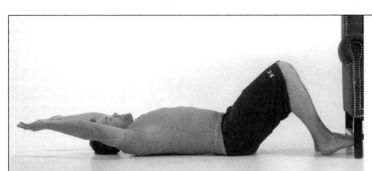

5 Lie flat on the floor in starting position.

Intermediate Sit-Ups (elbow hits)

1 Lie flat on the floor with arms overhead, knees bent at a 90-degree angle, and feet tucked under a sofa or heavy armchair.

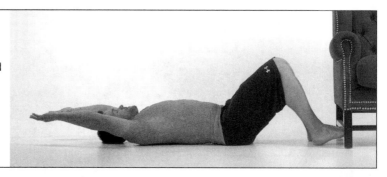

2 Swing arms forward and sit up, crunching forcefully with your abdominal muscles.

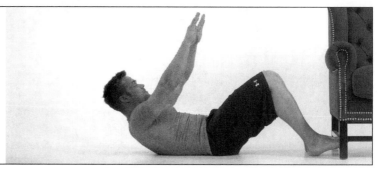

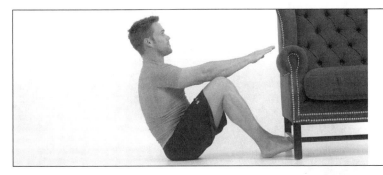

3 Hit the inside of your knees with your elbows to mark the top of the rep.

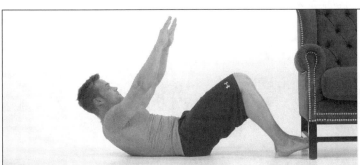

4 Return to the lying-down position to complete the rep.

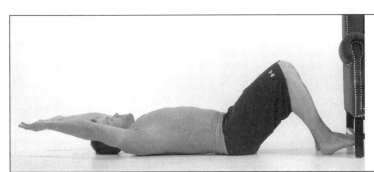

5 Lie flat on the floor in starting position.

Advanced Sit-Ups (military style)

1 Lie flat on the floor with hands clasped behind your head, elbows out to the sides, knees bent at a 90-degree angle, and feet tucked under a sofa or heavy armchair.

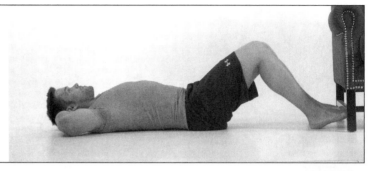

2 Sit up and crunch forcefully with your abdominal muscles.

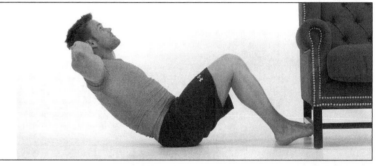

3 Your farthest range of motion marks the top of the rep. Your torso should reach nearly vertical.

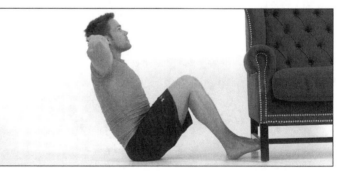

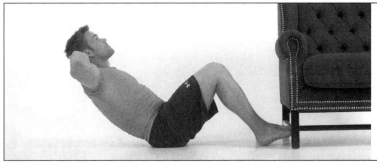

4 Return to the lying-down position to complete the rep.

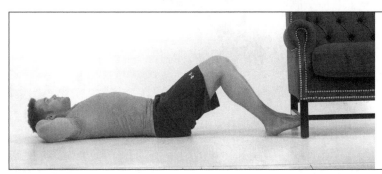

5 Lie flat on the floor in starting position.

DON'TS

DON'T

Don't round your back at the top of the sit-up.

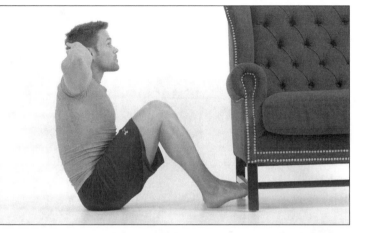

DON'T

Don't pull your chin to your chest during the sit-up. Keep the chin pointed toward the ceiling.

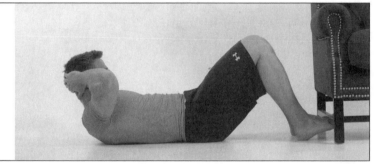

DON'T

Don't hold your breath during the sit-up! Focus on your breathing techniques. When learning the sit-up, you should naturally exhale during the upward motion.

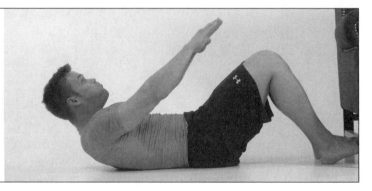

For a sit-up to count, your shoulder blades must be touching the floor at the beginning of each rep.

Push-Ups
Beginner Push-Ups (cobras or baby-ups)

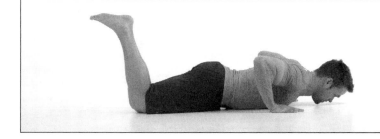

1 Lie flat on the floor on your belly, feet together, hands tucked underneath your shoulders, palms down, facing forward, and elbows at a 45-degree angle.

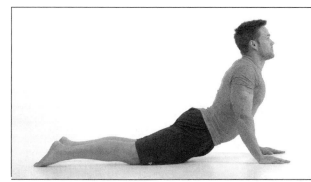

2 Full lockout of your elbows (straight arms) marks the top of the rep.

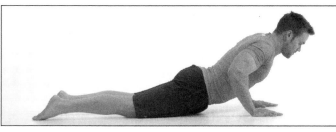

3 Return to the lying-down position to complete the rep.

Intermediate Push-Ups (knee-ups)

1 Lie flat on the floor on your belly, feet together, hands tucked underneath your shoulders, palms down, facing forward, and elbows at a 45-degree angle.

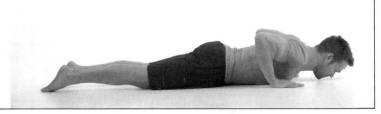

2 Press forcefully against the floor with your arms, keeping your abs tight and your body rigid like a board from your shoulders to your knees.

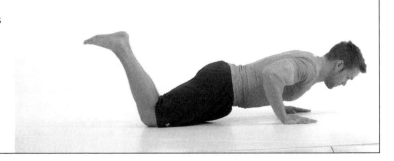

3 Full lockout of your elbows (straight arms) marks the top of the rep.

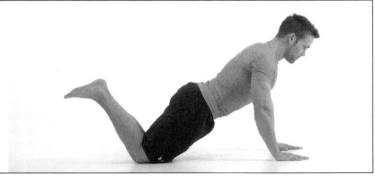

Advanced Push-Ups (military style)

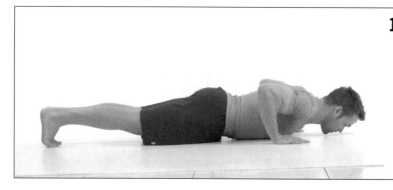

1 Lie flat on the floor on your belly, feet together with toes pointed down, hands tucked underneath your shoulders palms down, facing forward, and elbows at a 45-degree angle.

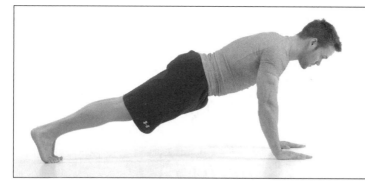

2 Press forcefully against the floor with your arms, keeping your abs tight and your body rigid like a board from your shoulders to your toes.

3 Full lockout of your elbows (straight arms) marks the top of the rep.

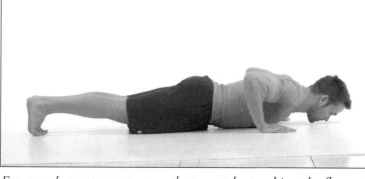

4 Return to the lying-down position to complete the rep.

125

For a push-up to count, your chest must be touching the floor at the beginning of the rep.

FOCUS ON

Focus on keeping your hands
underneath the shoulders and
elbows at a 45-degree angle.

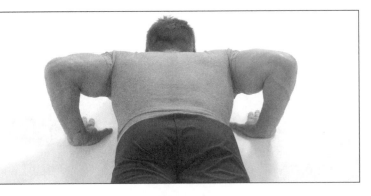

Keep abs tight and body rigid as
you press upward.

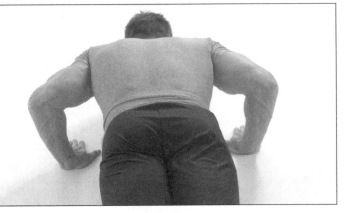

Lock the elbows out to mark the
top of the rep.

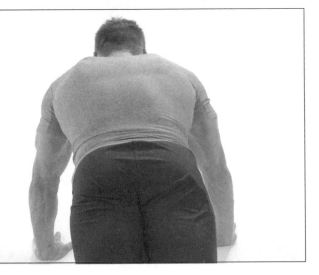

DON'TS

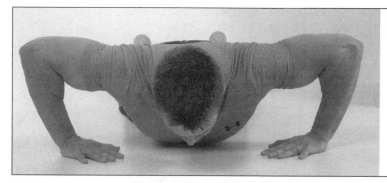

DON'T

Don't allow your elbows to point outward and your hands to point inward during the push-up.

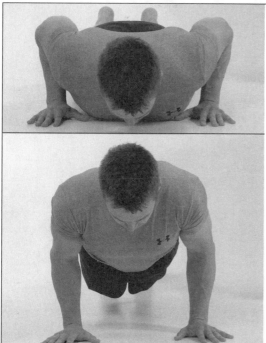

DON'T

Don't allow your elbows to tuck in too tight. Although this is a great press, let's focus on the regular push-up first!

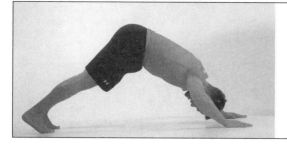

DON'T

Don't allow your body to pike upward or to "dive" into the push-up. The hands should stay directly under the shoulders and along the chest line.

Squats
Beginner Squats

1 Stand tall with your weight on
your heels, knees slightly bent,
feet apart at shoulder width, and
toes pointed slightly outward.

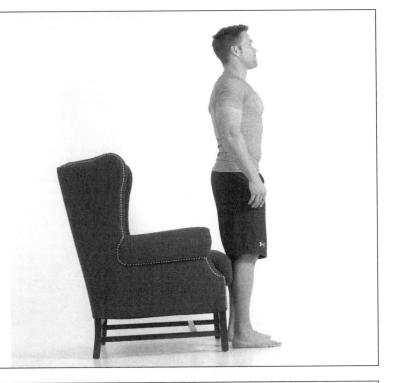

2 Keeping your weight on your
heels, lower your glutes (butt)
down and out. If necessary, use a
sofa or chair armrest to support
yourself and keep your balance.

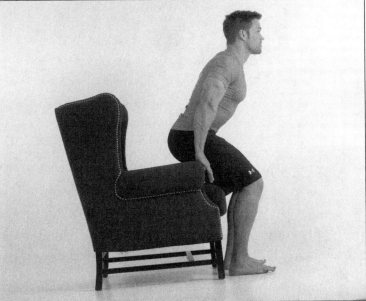

Beginner Squats

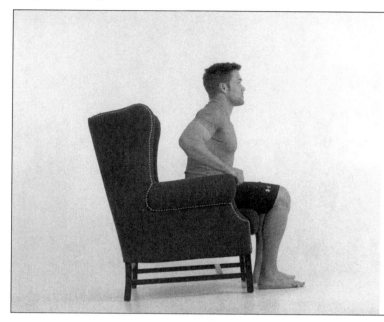

3 Full seated-position (knees at a 90-degree angle) with your weight shifted to your glutes marks the bottom of the rep.

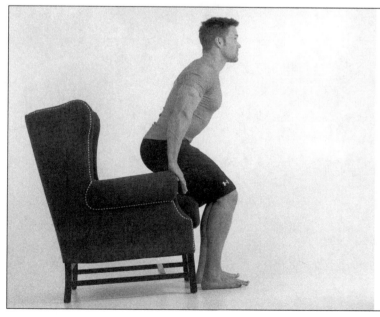

4 Press forcefully through your heels back to the standing tall position to complete the rep.

Beginner Squats

5 Stand tall in starting position.

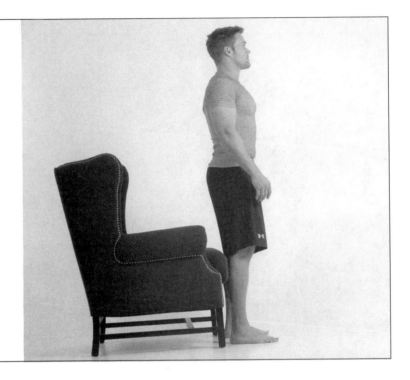

At the bottom of the squat, knees should track outward, in the direction of the toes, and weight should remain on the heels. Use an armrest to help support your bodyweight throughout the movement.

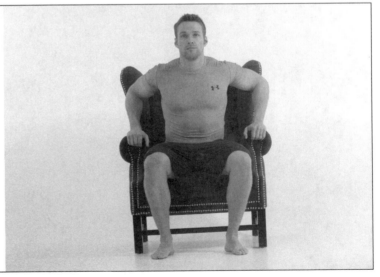

Intermediate Squats

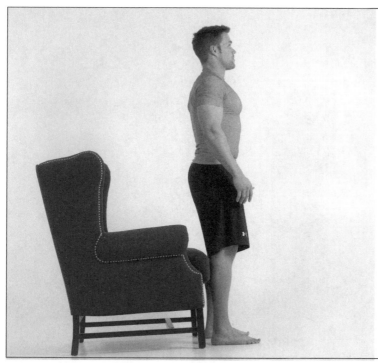

1 Stand tall with your weight on your heels, knees slightly bent, feet apart at shoulder width, and toes pointed slightly outward.

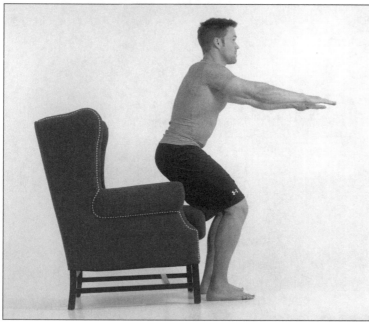

2 Keeping your weight on your heels, lower your hips down and back. Extend your arms forward as a counterbalance.

Intermediate Squats

3 Gently touch your glutes (butt) to a chair or sofa seat to mark the bottom of the rep.

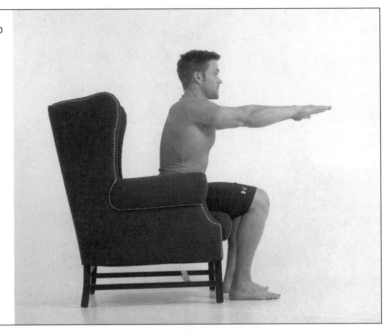

4 Press forcefully through your heels back to the standing tall position to complete the rep.

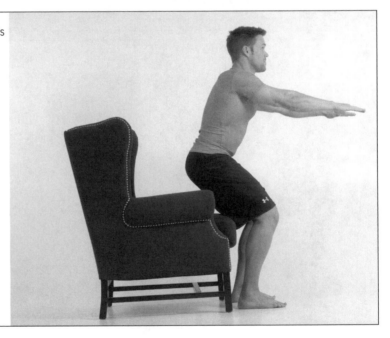

Intermediate Squats

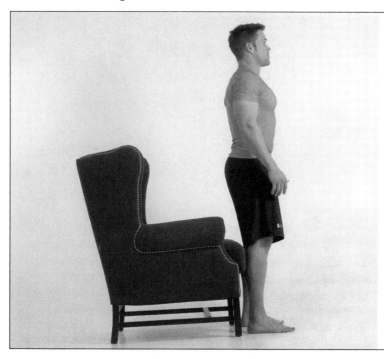

5 Stand tall in starting position.

FOCUS

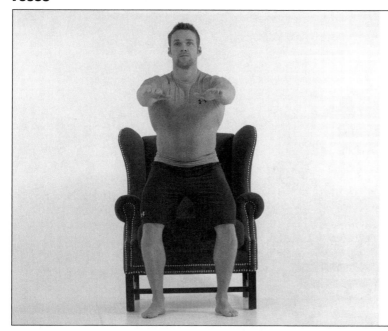

Use the arms as a counterbalance when lowering your backside to a seated position.

Advanced Squats (military style)

1 Stand tall with your weight on your heels, knees slightly bent, feet apart at shoulder width, and toes pointed slightly outward.

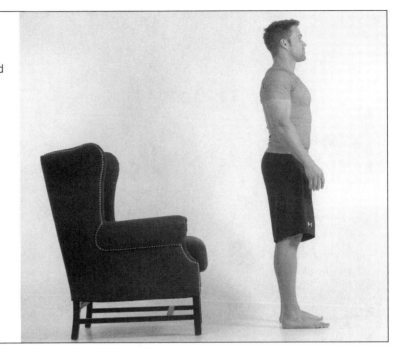

2 Keeping your weight on your heels, lower your hips down and back. Extend your arms forward as a counterbalance.

134

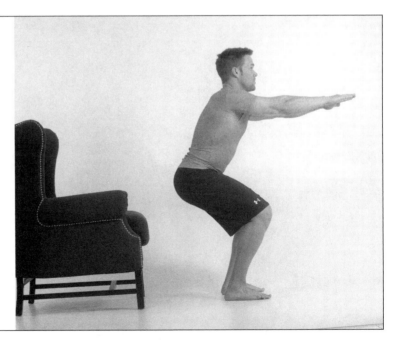

Advanced Squats (military style)

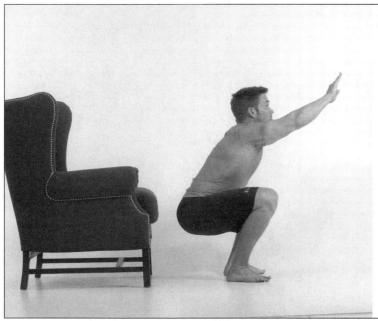

3 Drop the crease at your hip below your knees to mark the bottom of the rep.

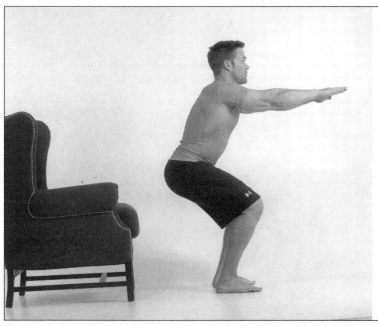

4 Press forcefully through your heels back to the standing tall position to complete the rep.

Advanced Squats (military style)

5 Stand tall in starting position.

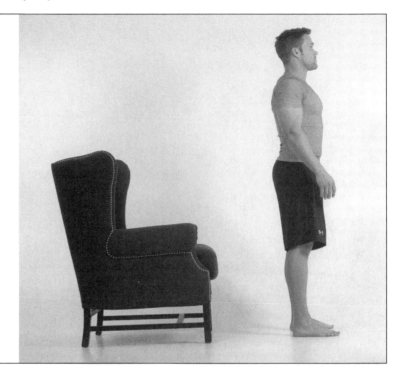

FOCUS ON

At the bottom of the motion, hands should be extended outward and upward, keeping the chest up, with weight shifted back onto the heels. Knees should be tracking in the direction of the toes.

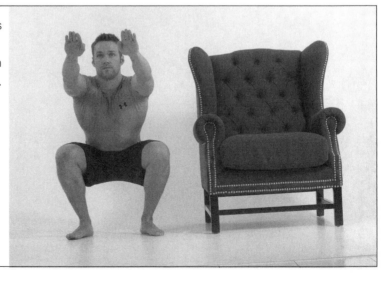

FOCUS ON

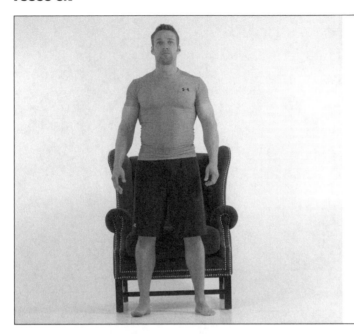

Focus on standing with the heels shoulder-width, and toes pointed gently outward.

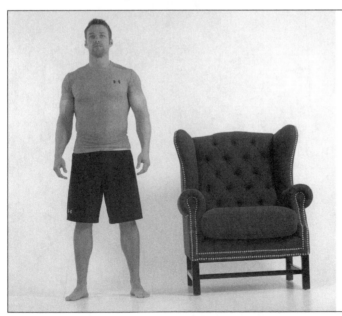

For the advanced squat, be sure to stand away from a sofa or chair.

For a squat to count, your knees and hips must be fully extended at the beginning of the rep (a slight bend in the knee is allowed).

DON'TS

DON'T

Don't knock your knees inward during the squat. Aggressively keep them in line with the direction of the toes.

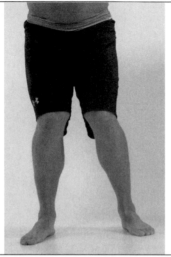

DON'T

Don't rise up onto your toes. Aggressively keep your weight shifted backward, heels planted firmly on the ground.

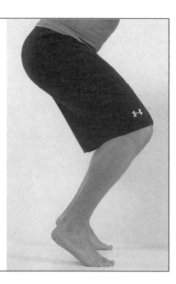

DON'T

Do not allow your shoulders to round as you reach forward. Aggressively keep your chest up and out.

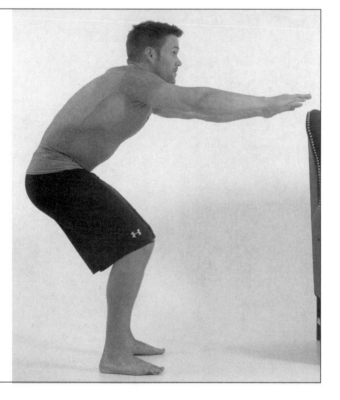

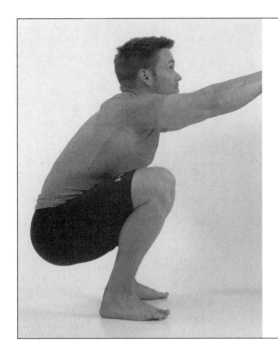

DON'T

Don't drop too far into the squat, so
that your lower back rounds.

MAXIMIZING **YOUR SHAPERS**

No two ways about it: Your body is going to challenge you when you do your shapers. Why else are they called workouts? It takes work—determination, energy, calories—to make your muscles grow. But you can take control of your body with your mind. Here's how to start each day with a victory over your machine:

- *Put your mind in the right place.*
  Focus on your muscles and bones in motion and keep your mind there.

- *Separate your breathing.*
  Don't breathe at the tempo of the movement. If you're moving at a faster tempo, breathe at a slower tempo. If you're moving at a slower tempo, breathe at a faster tempo. Always be aware of your breath.

- *Separate your mind.*
  From the outside, feel the physical stress your body is experiencing, and observe its performance from an objective standpoint. Whether you're doing a sprint, endurance, or shape & size shaper, ride your body through the physical challenge. Focus on the separation of your body and your breathing. It's pretty trippy.

- *Conquer your fear.*
  As your body reaches the point when you feel it can't do anymore, you'll reach a climax moment. This is when fear comes pouring in. The voice inside your head gets so loud you can't ignore it. Perhaps you're about to start panic breathing during a sprint shaper. Perhaps your muscles are reaching a high-intensity burn during an endurance circuit. Perhaps you're shaking during a shape & size shaper. This is where people often give up. But it's also the point where you have an incredible opportunity to conquer your fear and break a mental barrier. Your body, your machine, will try to get you to hold your breath. Don't let it happen. Breathe, breathe, breathe! Only through good breathing will you be physically and mentally able to explore beyond the barrier.

- *Go past the point of climax.*
  Be curious, not fearful, about what lies beyond that point. No one can describe that transcendence, and only you can feel it. In this moment, you'll get a fleeting glimpse of your true potential and your true power. You'll reach a point where you no longer think about the toiling of your heart, lungs, muscles, and joints. The flash lasts only a second, but the afterglow stays with you for days, months and even years . . . and lets you strive toward awesomeness. You're gonna love this ride!

SHREDDERS

Are you ready to burn some fat? Yes! Let's crank up your body's furnace by doing some shredders. These cardio workouts get your muscles blazing and take your metabolic rate to astronomical levels. Shredders turn your body into a monster fat-burning machine. The more you shred, the more body fat you burn. The more time you dedicate to shredding, the faster you'll reach your weight-loss goal.

Shredders are cardio intervals of walking, jogging, rowing, bicycle riding, rope jumping, or other exercises that get your heart pumping and speed the flow of oxygenated blood to your organs. Studies have proven that intervals—cycling between high- and low-intensity cardiovascular exercise—generate a much more effective and long-lasting metabolic spike and afterburn than steady-state cardio alone. Your body will burn calories for a longer period of time following your workout. The brief period of slightly higher-intensity exercise in each circuit raises your metabolism for several hours afterward. Not only do you burn a lot of calories while you exercise, your body stays revved up for a long time.

Your metabolism isn't the only thing that benefits. Cardiovascular intervals boost endurance and stamina. Cardio also increases delivery of oxygen to your tissues, improves digestion, strengthens your heart, and does lots of other good things.

The best cardiovascular exercises are those you enjoy most. If you force yourself to do any particular exercise, you won't be at it for long. So if you know you love to run on a treadmill, swim, or cross-country ski, go for it and have fun. If you aren't sure which cardiovascular activities you like most, I invite you to experiment. For the purpose of shredding, it's easiest to choose exercises that you can do on your own. Try:

- Walking, jogging, or running

- Stair climbing or rope jumping

- Bicycle riding, mountain biking, or spinning

- Swimming, cross-country skiing, or rowing

- Working out on the cardio equipment at a gym

THE MORE THE MERRIER

If you're not accustomed to cardiovascular exercise, start out easy. It's important to give your body enough time to adjust to its new routine. However fit you are when you come to The Carb-Cycle Solution—as a beginner, intermediate, or advanced exerciser—start at your comfort level, and work up from there.

Each shredder is six minutes long. If you're physically able, begin with five shredders daily for 30 awesome, fat-burning minutes of exercise. But if you have been sedentary for years and are just learning to move again, you should start with just two full six-minute shredders at a relatively light intensity. This will take just 12 minutes, but the benefits will last for days.

Increase the length and intensity of your exercise by one six-minute shredder per week until you can circuit comfortably for at least five shredders—30 minutes. Once you are at five shredders daily, you'll start adding more shredders to your workouts. This gradual increase in the amount of exercise you do daily is called *progressive overload*. Fitness professionals of all stripes use this method in all their clients' transformations for continued and rapid fat loss.

DOUBLE SPIKE

Don't have 30 minutes open in your schedule? You can split your shredder workout into two daily sessions. For example, if you have six shredders to complete, you could do three in the afternoon and three in the evening. Exercising twice a day causes your metabolism to spike *twice*. By the end of the day, you'll burn more calories with two exercise sessions than with one, even if your total workout time is the same. Many of my clients split their shredders into two sessions just to maximize the metabolic afterburn for the fastest results! Exercising twice a day might be inconvenient for you, but if you can schedule it in, by all means do it!

SHREDDER INTENSITY

During each shredder, or cardio interval, you circuit the intensity of your exercise according to a defined pattern to maximize fat burning. Shredders circuit your exercise intensity through three levels: light, moderate, and high—for example, climbing stairs slowly, faster, and as fast as you can. It's the best way to do cardio if your goal is to lose weight.

In the fitness world, cardiovascular exercise intensity is often gauged by a measure called perceived exertion (PE). Perceived exertion is exactly what it sounds like: the level of exertion at which you perceive you're working. The greater your fitness level, the more exercise you can do at a given level of perceived exertion. To make it easy for you, I've put together a perceived exertion scale with levels between 6 and 10, including the physical markers of breathing and ease of conversation, which help you gauge your intensity level.

CARB DAYS

PE LEVEL	INTENSITY	TALK TEST
6	Light	unbroken conversation, breathing easy
7	Moderate	unbroken conversation, breathing heavy
8	Brisk	conversation broken, three to four words at a time
9	Fast	conversation broken, only single words
10	All-Out	cannot talk, panic breathing

Cycle through each shredder based on your PE levels:

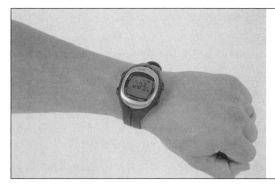

• Three minutes at low intensity (e.g., riding your bike on a flat trail)

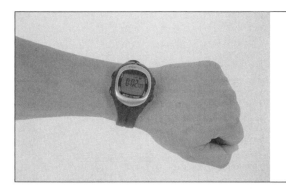

• Two minutes at moderate intensity (e.g., riding fast on a flat trail)

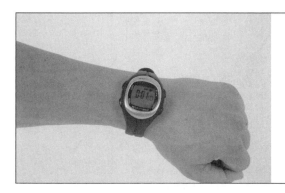

• One minute at high intensity (e.g., climbing a hill on your bike)
Altogether, this equals one six-minute shredder.

YOUR SHREDDER CALENDAR

There are two components to your shredder calendar: the number of shredders you do and the intensity at which you do them.

Guess what? Within a couple weeks of starting your shredder regimen, your body will adapt to your 30-minute workout. So you need to bump things up for increased fat-loss results. Step up your workout by one six-minute shredder every two weeks to keep fat burning maximized at every single session.

During each three-month period you're on The Carb-Cycle Solution, you add to the number of shredders you do each day, from five shredders a day in Week One, to 10 shredders a day in Week 12. When you complete Phase One—the first 90 days of your program—you start the process over again for 90 days in Phase Two, building from five shredders a day at the beginning to 10 shredders a day at the end. Continue this pattern for as many 90-day phases as you need to reach your goal weight.

With each successive 90-day phase, your PE levels increase. In Phase One, your six-minute shredder has three minutes of low-intensity exercise at PE 6, two minutes of moderate-intensity exercise at PE 7, and one minute of high-intensity exercise at PE 8. For Phase Two, you crank your power to PE 7, PE 8, and PE 9, respectively. Your exertion climbs one PE level per each 90-day period.

Here's how the first two phases pan out.

SHREDDER PHASES

SHREDDER PHASE 1: 90 DAYS	COUNT / DURATION	INTENSITY		
		LOW	MODERATE	HIGH
Weeks 1–2	5 shredders, 30 minutes	PE 6	PE 7	PE 8
Weeks 3–4	6 shredders, 36 minutes	PE 6	PE 7	PE 8
Weeks 5–6	7 shredders, 42 minutes	PE 6	PE 7	PE 8
Weeks 7–8	8 shredders, 48 minutes	PE 6	PE 7	PE 8
Weeks 9–10	9 shredders, 54 minutes	PE 6	PE 7	PE 8
Weeks 11–12	10 shredders, 60 minutes	PE 6	PE 7	PE 8
SHREDDER PHASE 2: 90 DAYS	COUNT / DURATION	INTENSITY		
		LOW	MODERATE	HIGH
Weeks 13–14	5 shredders, 30 minutes	PE 7	PE 8	PE 9
Weeks 15–16	6 shredders, 36 minutes	PE 7	PE 8	PE 9
Weeks 17–18	7 shredders, 42 minutes	PE 7	PE 8	PE 9
Weeks 19–20	8 shredders, 48 minutes	PE 7	PE 8	PE 9
Weeks 21–22	9 shredders, 54 minutes	PE 7	PE 8	PE 9
Weeks 23–24	10 shredders, 60 minutes	PE 7	PE 8	PE 9

VARIETY IS THE SPICE OF SHREDDING

Just as it's important to increase the intensity and duration of your shredder workouts, it's important to change the type of exercise as well. Your body will adapt to whatever kind of cardio exercise you do. If you love spinning, rollerblading, or mountain biking shredders, more power to you. However, if you're starting to feel stale and you want to switch things up, start exploring new options!

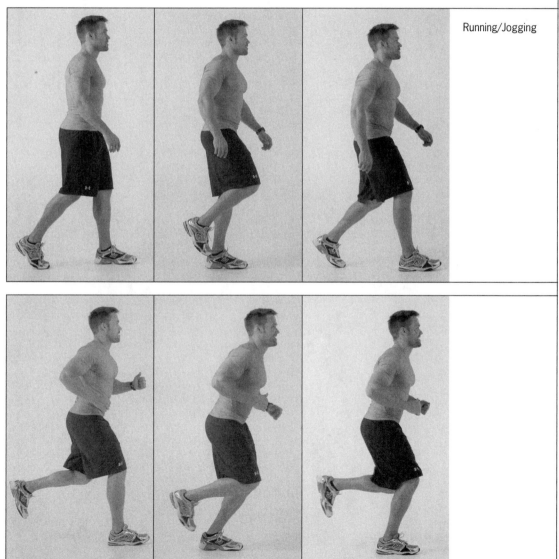

Running/Jogging

145

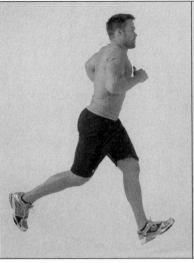
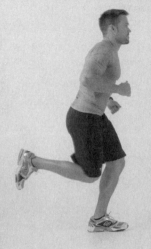
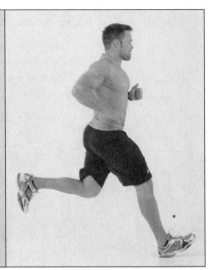

Jumping Rope

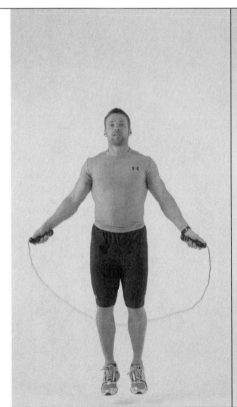
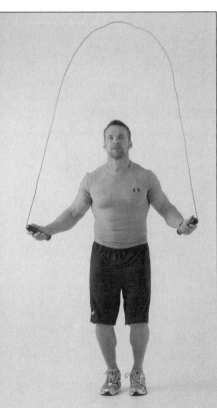

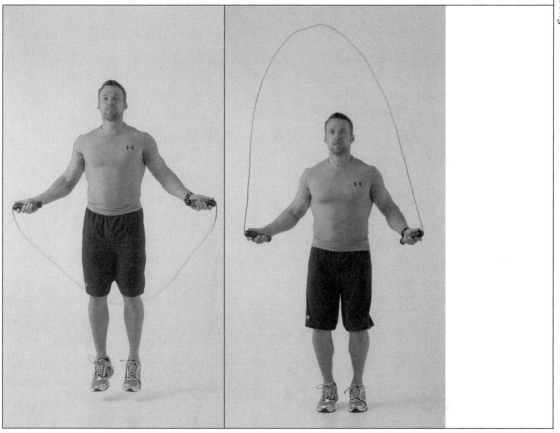

You'll get your best shredder results if you alternate your activities. In fact, the more variety there is in your workout, the better your fitness level. If you always walk, that's fine. But if you alternate walking with rowing and cycling, that's superb. You'll be using your muscles in different ways, so your body won't become too efficient at any particular kind of exercise. You know by now that when your body doesn't adapt, you lose weight faster.

In the athletic world, physiologists and exercise scientists have found evidence that training programs consistently plateau. When an athlete follows an unchanging exercise regimen, his or her performance plateaus after a very short period of time (usually within a few weeks). To overcome this, the best training programs are based on periodization, the practice of constantly changing the type of exercise as well as the workload, intensity, duration, and rest periods to prevent a performance plateau.

147

DON'T HURT **YOURSELF**

As you embrace your new lifestyle and exercise routine, one thing I can guarantee is that you'll experience the occasional physical setback. It happens! DO NOT let it slow your momentum. Blisters, chafing, joint discomfort, swelling, and plantar fasciitis (pain and swelling on the sole of the foot) can crop up along the way. Be prepared, anticipate the setbacks, and have the right tools ready when you need them. Don't let any obstacle get in your way.

TOOLS FOR INJURY PREVENTION	
Blisters	Powder Dry socks, Moleskin
Chafing	Powder, Ointments, Petroleum jelly
Fungus	Alternating your socks Alternating your shoes
Joints	Knee brace/patellar band, Two pairs of heavy-duty walking shoes, Ice packs, Glucosamine & chondroitin
Plantar Fasciitis	Special shoes, New shoes every three months, Athletic tape, Shoe inserts
Swelling	Ice packs, Epsom salt baths, Compression shorts, Compression stockings
Comfort	Dry, loose clothing
Entertainment and Tracking	MP3 player, Heart rate monitor, Pedometer

REST DAYS

Losing weight is taxing on your body. As you work hard through the week, you stress your body. When it's stressed, your body releases the hormone cortisol into your bloodstream. Cortisol triggers the storage of body fat (especially around the abdomen), so you want to clear this hormone out of your system ASAP! You must give your body and mind one day a week to rest and relax. This will reduce your cortisol levels, allowing your body to recover and prepare for more weight loss in the coming week.

The Carb-Cycle Solution designates Sunday as your rest day. If your schedule doesn't allow you to rest on Sunday, choose another rest day as your schedule permits, but make sure to take one on the same day every week. It's imperative that you don't exercise on this day—no shapers and no shredders!

CHAPTER 13:
PUTTING IT ALL TOGETHER

You can lose weight on The Carb-Cycle Solution by carb cycling alone, but your results increase exponentially if you add exercise. Weight loss speeds up dramatically, and your overall health and fitness levels soar. By coordinating high-carb and low-carb days with shapers and shredders, you burn more calories, build more muscle mass, boost your metabolism, and lose weight faster.

During your 7-Day Carb Cycles, do shredders for six days to maximize fat-burning and shapers on your three low-carb days when you have extra carb energy built up (from the preceding high-carb day) to power your muscles. During your slingshot weeks, do shapers and shredders on alternate days for six days. After six days of exercise in both carb cycle and slingshot weeks, *it's essential that you take a day to rest* so your body can recover. All you have to do on day seven is relax!

THE CARB-CYCLE SOLUTION CALENDAR

Here's how to combine carb cycling with shapers and shredders for an ideal weight-loss week. The chart details Phase One of your program; Phase Two is much the same, except your shredder intensities increase to PE 7/8/9.

PHASE ONE: **THE FIRST 90 DAYS**

MONTH 1

	SUNDAY	MONDAY	TUESDAY	WEDNESDAY	THURSDAY	FRIDAY	SATURDAY
7-Day Carb Cycles	Free / High-Carb	Low-Carb	High-Carb	Low-Carb	High-Carb	Low-Carb	High-Carb
Shapers Weeks 1–3	Rest	Sprint Shaper		Endurance Shaper		Shape & Size Shaper	**Weigh-In**
Shredders Weeks 1–2,	Rest	5	5	5	5	5	5
Shredders Week 3	Rest	6	6	6	6	6	6
Slingshot	High-Carb	High-Carb	High-Carb	High-Carb	High-Carb	High-Carb	High-Carb
Shapers Week 4	Rest	Sprint Shaper		Endurance Shaper		Shape & Size Shaper	**Weigh-In**
Shredders Week 4	Rest	6	6	6	6	6	6

MONTH 2

	SUNDAY	MONDAY	TUESDAY	WEDNESDAY	THURSDAY	FRIDAY	SATURDAY
7-Day Carb Cycles	Free / High-Carb	Low-Carb	High-Carb	Low-Carb	High-Carb	Low-Carb	High-Carb
Shapers Weeks 5–7	Rest	Sprint Shaper		Endurance Shaper		Shape & Size Shaper	**Weigh-In**
Shredders Weeks 5–6	Rest	7	7	7	7	7	7
Shredders Week 7	Rest	8	8	8	8	8	8
Slingshot	High-Carb	High-Carb	High-Carb	High-Carb	High-Carb	High-Carb	High-Carb
Shapers Week 8	Rest	Sprint Shaper		Endurance Shaper		Shape & Size Shaper	**Weigh-In**
Shredders Week 8	Rest	8	8	8	8	8	8

MONTH 3

	SUNDAY	MONDAY	TUESDAY	WEDNESDAY	THURSDAY	FRIDAY	SATURDAY
7-Day Carb Cycles	Free / High-Carb	Low-Carb	High-Carb	Low-Carb	High-Carb	Low-Carb	High-Carb
Shapers Weeks 9–11	Rest	Sprint Shaper		Endurance Shaper		Shape & Size Shaper	**Weigh-In**
Shredders Weeks 9–10	Rest	9	9	9	9	9	9
Shredders Week 11	Rest	10	10	10	10	10	10
Slingshot	High-Carb	High-Carb	High-Carb	High-Carb	High-Carb	High-Carb	High-Carb
Shapers Week 12	Rest	Sprint Shaper		Endurance Shaper		Shape & Size Shaper	**Weigh-In**
Shredders Week 12	Rest	10	10	10	10	10	10

MOVING FORWARD: YOUR FIRST FOUR WEEKS

When you launch into The Carb-Cycle Solution, you'll soon see exciting changes in your body. Some people start to lose weight immediately, while for others, weight loss begins after two to four weeks on the program. Every single person whom I have guided through this program has been successful, but some take longer than others. Even though all bodies function according to the same scientific principles, they respond to diet and exercise differently. Many factors are at play. The rate at which you lose weight has to do primarily with how far overweight you are at the start of the program. The more weight you need to lose, the faster your body can lose it.

Your previous lifestyle habits, your age, your genes, and any other quirks your body might have can affect how quickly you reach your goal. If you're a 60-year-old woman and you want to lose five pounds, your results will be less dramatic over several weeks than the progress experienced by a 35-year-old who needs to drop 100 pounds.

Over the course of the next several weeks, you'll learn to listen to your body. You'll *feel* when you're losing weight. You'll *feel* when you boost your metabolism. You'll *feel* when you retain and flush water. You'll *feel* every ounce of food you eat. You'll *feel* when your body begins to adapt to changes. Your body will always talk to you, and you'll learn how to speak your own language, discovering how to interpret, understand, and appreciate your transformation over the weeks to come.

PROGRESS: WEEK ONE

Welcome to your first 7-Day Carb Cycle! You're beginning to understand the importance of alternating between high-carb days without shapers and low-carb days with shapers. You can also sense the wisdom of working six shredder days and one rest day into your week.

At the beginning of The Carb-Cycle Solution, you may notice that your energy levels can drop slightly after meals on your high-carb days. This is because you're eating food that requires a lot of energy to digest and assimilate. Within a week, though, your energy level on high-carb days will come right back up with your metabolism. Before you know it, you'll be bouncing off the walls, just in time for your low-carb days! On your low-carb days, your energy level may drop throughout the day, but you'll be burning fat like crazy and your energy will return tomorrow, a high-carb day.

Some people may experience the opposite pattern when they first start the program, with low energy on high-carb days and high energy on low-carb days.

But as you progress through the program, this tendency will reverse when your body adjusts to your new, healthier eating habits.

The Carb-Cycle Solution is about learning to listen to your body. As you groove into the program and your energy level climbs and drops on alternating high- and low-carb days, embrace the differences you feel! This is your body talking to you, telling you that it's beginning to make some adjustments. The next several weeks will be very rewarding.

This first 7-Day Carb Cycle is always the most difficult when it comes to adopting new lifestyle patterns. Learning how to prepare your food in bulk and carry meals with you is usually one of the biggest challenges. For speedy and nearly effortless food and recipe ideas, check out the "Quick and Easy On-the-Go Foods" section in Chapter 9 and the recipes in Chapter 15. You'll quickly learn shortcuts and tricks for prepping your meals, so just stick with it—it gets so much easier!

PROGRESS: WEEK TWO

Give yourself a pat on the back for sticking with The Carb-Cycle Solution. Altering your lifestyle is especially difficult when you first get started, but you're doing it! Now that you've gotten through the first 7-Day Carb Cycle, you should be noticing a few things about your body. You probably have lots of energy on high-carb days and may feel slightly lethargic on low-carb days. That's exactly as it should be. (Remember, if you need a little extra kick on low-carb days, you may add some light caffeine from sources like green tea. It can help significantly with your energy level and give your metabolism a bit of a boost as well. If you're a heavy caffeine user and prefer coffee, that's okay. But first, consult with your doctor about caffeine use.)

If you don't notice the scale going down, but you're doing the daily workouts, you're most likely going through recomposition: gaining muscle and losing fat at the same time. During this process, you'll likely lose inches but remain the same weight until your body gains fat-burning muscle from resistance exercise. Proper nutrition gives your muscles a chance to reach their full potential. Once they do, they'll help you lose a lot of fat. Most of my clients go through recomposition for two to four weeks before they start losing weight—fast. It's truly a beautiful thing.

You should only weigh yourself once this week, but if you can't stay off the scale, you'll notice that your weight fluctuates by a few pounds a day. People who are really heavy can see even greater differences. What's going on? You're gaining and losing water weight, a good sign that your body is responding to the 7-Day Carb Cycles. Retaining and then flushing water is a natural part of adjusting to carb cycling. Don't try to fiddle with the program to chase after weight loss: You'll only become frustrated. Go with the flow!

Now that you've gotten used to doing your shaper workouts, focus on keeping your form as precise as possible. The better your form, the more intense the workout will be. Don't rush your workout, compromising form to complete maximum reps. Follow the instructions in Chapter 12 to get the most from your exercise.

It's the second week of your shredder workouts, so you may feel you can bump up your intensity a bit. Remember to stay at perceived exertion (PE) levels of 6, 7, and 8. There's no need to work harder than that right now. We want to save those higher intensities for later phases if we need them! Trust your own inner guidance system as you monitor your exercise intensity.

You and your body are still getting used to your new habits. As with all change, the first days are the hardest. When you're accustomed to your new lifestyle, you'll have formed healthier habits that will lead to a fresh, healthier you. Hang in there through this period of adjustment. Your rewards are just around the corner!

PHOTO **OPPORTUNITY**

While you're remaking your body, your eyes will play tricks on you. Remember that what you see in the mirror is NOT reality. A great way to track your progress and validate your success is to take pictures. Photos will give you an objective view of your transformation. Plus, it's fun to see how far you've come! Here are a few photo pointers to help you out:

Tip #1: Keep in mind that these pics are just for you. You don't have to share them with anyone else, unless you want to.

Tip #2: For your photo session, wear clothing that allows you to see every part of your transforming body. Since you're the only one who'll be looking at the pics, lose the turtleneck. Shorts and a sports bra are perfect.

Tip #3: Shoot a few pictures from different angles. Front and side-profile shots are the most popular.

Tip #4: Take pictures every week. Even though you won't be able to see the gradual changes as they happen, when you line up the pictures next to each other after a few weeks, you'll be blown away at how much you've changed!

Tip #5: Use the photos as daily reminders of your achievement by placing copies in one or more visible spots. Try inside your fridge, on your bathroom mirror, in a favorite part of your room, or at the bottom of a drawer that you use a lot. If you're REALLY proud of the new you, use the photos as your screen saver!

Have fun clicking away! It will give you a whole new admiration for your incredible body.

PROGRESS: WEEK THREE

Great job! You're now two weeks into The Carb-Cycle Solution, and you can take a step back to evaluate what's happening with your body.

During your third 7-Day Carb Cycle, the ups and downs in your energy level should be in full swing, with high energy on high-carb days and low energy on low-carb days. You might also be retaining and flushing water in a predictable pattern, feeling slightly bloated after high-carb days and leaner after low-carb days. These cycles are normal—in fact, they're a good sign that your body isn't adapting to the program and holding onto extra weight. You're controlling your body so that it sheds those unwanted pounds.

If you haven't lost weight yet, you may need to make some tweaks to the program to start seeing progress. Check out the "Troubleshooting" section at the end of Chapter 9 for tips.

You may have become more sensitive to the foods and drinks you consume. Many of my clients, for example, notice that their daily cup of coffee sends them through the roof. Any such changes you see are a sign that you're well on your way to clearing your body of the bad stuff you used to feed it. Our bodies are supposed to be sensitive, and we're supposed to be tuned in to what they tell us. If you're regaining this ability, congratulations! It means you're becoming healthier.

Your shaper workouts should be feeling more comfortable. Throughout the movements, play with different timing and exertion to make them as challenging as possible. Keep your form correct, and listen to your muscles. Follow the rules, and maximize those reps!

By now, your body has most likely adjusted to five daily shredders, and you've found that they're getting easier, right? That's why it's time to bump up to six shredders a day to maximize fat-burning. Keep your intensity to PE levels 6, 7, and 8, and burn away.

You're learning to incorporate carb cycling into your lifestyle. Once you set the pattern, you can and will lose weight—however and whenever you choose. Again, well done. Keep up the good work, and enjoy your success!

PROGRESS: WEEK FOUR

Great job on your dedication to The Carb-Cycle Solution! You've followed the 7-Day Carb Cycle for three full weeks now and are probably witnessing some big changes. It's time to reset your body with a slingshot week. Prepare for seven high-carb days in a row.

Even if you've been noticing substantial drops on the scale every week, it's still important to slingshot this week, just to keep your metabolism guessing. The reset will ensure that you continue to drop pounds next week, when you go back to carb cycling. While slingshotting, it's common to experience slight water retention and a slowdown on the scale due to the high-carb diet, but many people do see continued weight loss. Either way, trust in the process, and reset your body for next week. You'll be glad you did!

This week should bring a substantial increase in your energy level and mental alertness. You should also experience stellar strength, endurance, and stamina during your shaper workouts because you're getting so many carbs—your muscles are all fueled up! Enjoy the high energy levels and incredible performance, and get ready to drop back into another 7-Day Carb Cycle next week to continue your weight-loss journey.

I'm so proud of you for hanging in there for this long. Keep up the fantastic work, and if you're not already, you'll soon be looking in the mirror at a whole new you.

CHAPTER 14:

THE LONG-TERM LIFESTYLE FOR WEIGHT-LOSS MAINTENANCE

Congratulations! You've reached your goal weight by following The Carb-Cycle Solution. Far more important than dropping your extra pounds, however, you have undergone a life transformation. You have purified your body, restored your sensitivity to nutrition, increased your metabolism, revealed your beautiful, sculpted body, and gotten in the best shape of your life.

THE MAINTENANCE MINDSET

Take some time to think about how you've changed. Acknowledge and appreciate that you did this yourself! Now you know how to create your dream body. Now you understand how the process works. You've taken control of your body and your life, and you now have the knowledge you need to transform your mind and your body whenever you wish, for the rest of your life.

To deepen your commitment to maintaining your gorgeous body, remind yourself of your many successes along the path to fabulousness. Small victories along your journey might have taken many forms:

Dropping a clothing size every couple of weeks

Notching your belt to smaller and smaller sizes

Watching your fat pants fall off

Buying suspenders to keep your pants up

Fitting into one leg of your old jeans

Slipping into your high school clothes

Seeing your fat rings melt away

Glimpsing your collarbone for the first time

Noticing the veins in your forearms and biceps

Removing your seatbelt extender

Taking up one seat in the theater or airplane

Not worrying about breaking any chairs you sit in

Sitting in a restaurant booth again

Completing multiple shaper circuits

Running your first mile, 5k, 10k, half-marathon, or marathon

Going out in public without attracting unwanted attention

Receiving compliments from strangers

Helping family, friends, and loved ones achieve their weight-loss goals

MEASURING **YOUR SUCCESS**

One of the most wonderful gifts you can give yourself during your transformation is proof of your progress. Hard, objective facts make it difficult to deny your huge success. When you've reached your ideal weight, take your measurements. Compare these numbers to the measurements you took before starting the program: You've got solid proof of your achievement. You've made the transition to your true self and have enhanced your health and happiness. Celebrate!

Date: _____

Weight: _____

Clothing size: _____

Circumference Measurements:

Neck - Measure the circumference of your neck at the midpoint, around the Adam's apple.

_____ inches

Chest - Measure the circumference of your chest along the "nipple line." It's important to keep your arms at your side.

_____ inches

Waist - Measure the circumference of your waist at the narrowest point (usually at the navel).

_____ inches

Hips - Measure the circumference of your hips at the widest point (usually about 6 to 8 inches below your waist).

_____ inches

Thigh - Measure the circumference of your RIGHT thigh at a point about 8 inches above the knee.

_____ inches

There's nothing like proof positive to validate your accomplishment. Now's the time to celebrate by taking "after" pictures of yourself. It's a whole lot more fun to snap these pics than it was to commit your old self to film! Compare your fresh shots to your "before" pictures, and admire your transformation.

A RECIPE FOR LASTING SUCCESS

Now that you've reached your goal weight and shape, you'll certainly want to keep the beautiful body you've created. There's a very straightforward formula for maintaining fantastic fitness. Client after client of mine has followed this maintenance plan, and they're always thrilled and astonished that it actually works. If you're like my other clients, you'll be absolutely amazed at how simple it is to enjoy your wonderful achievement—forever.

For inspiration, remind yourself that if you choose to go back to your old eating habits and couch-potato lifestyle, your body will regress little by little to what it was when you began your weight-loss journey. Follow a few simple guidelines, and you should be able to stay at your ideal weight. If you ever find yourself gaining a few extra pounds, you now know how to lose them again quickly: Restart the 7-Day Carb Cycles and slingshots, and keep them going until you drop the pounds you've gained.

To maintain your ideal weight:

❏ *Eat five meals every day.*
  This should never change. Eat breakfast within 30 minutes of waking and every 3 hours afterward. Keep your metabolic furnace burning hot with five meals daily.

159

❏ *Eat a wide variety of foods.*

Choose all your food from the acceptable foods list (see Chapter 9). Eat lean meats and poultry, eggs, nonfat dairy, lots of fruits and vegetables, legumes, seeds, nuts, and healthy oils.

❏ *Eat a balanced diet.*

To maintain your weight, you won't need to carb cycle. For each meal, choose one portion of protein, one portion of carbs, one portion of fat, and unlimited veggies. This combination opens up a whole new world of recipes and meals. At first, the formula may seem to involve a significant amount of food—because it does. It's real, whole, healthy food with a lot of bulk but not a lot of calories! It's perfect for maintaining your beautiful new body.

❏ *Don't exceed your Carb-Cycle Solution portion sizes.*

All too often those portions creep back up. If you eat the correct Carb-Cycle Solution portion for you, you should be satisfied after each meal and have fantastic energy throughout the day.

❏ *Reward yourself once a day.*

By now, you may have curbed your cravings for unhealthy foods altogether. But if you still desire a sweet or salty treat, it's important to reward yourself every other day with a healthy treat that you enjoy, from a sugar-free drink to a portioned snack. Indulge in moderation, preferably earlier in the day. You may continue to have a free day at the end of your week (Option 1) OR cheat meals every other day (Option 2). Whatever works best for you!

❏ *Exercise.*

This should never change! Your body is made to move, so keep it moving with your morning shapers and daily shredders.

❏ *Drink lots of water.*

Stay hydrated throughout the day by drinking at least a gallon of water.

It's as simple as that!

INSPIRE OTHERS!

Sharing your accomplishments with the world can really energize you to stick with the maintenance program. I'd absolutely love to witness your success! I encourage you to send me your "before" and "after" pictures and to tell me how many pounds and inches you've lost. With your permission, I'd like to post your success on www.chrispowell.com so you can inspire others!

I invite you to contact me through my Web site. I welcome any thoughts you have about The Carb-Cycle Solution. I'm interested in knowing what parts of the program you like, what needs improvement, and how I can make it faster, easier, and more enjoyable in the future.

When you achieve amazing results with The Carb-Cycle Solution, please share your story with others, and help them discover the path to fast and permanent weight loss. It's a wonderful feeling to know you've opened the door for another person who seeks a happier, healthier life. Trust me. I feel it often, and that feeling motivates and inspires me every day.

Congratulations for proving to yourself that you have the inner strength and determination to change your life for the better. I'm proud of you. More important, however, is that you take this moment to be proud of yourself.

My most sincere wishes to you for a happy and healthy life!

Chris

CHAPTER 15:
RECIPES AND PORTIONS

Get ready for some tasty eating! The foods you're allowed to eat on The Carb-Cycle Solution are natural, delicious, and nutritious, so they'll help you stick to the program.

Suggested recipes for your breakfasts, snacks, lunches, and dinners are divided into high-carbohydrate and low-carbohydrate lists here. You'll find many wonderful ideas, but these aren't the only meals you can eat. Feel free to get creative and invent your own dishes. Using the approved Carb-Cycle Solution foods, you have limitless possibilities.

When creating the Carb-Cycle Solution, my goal was to develop a system that was not just scientifically sound, but also practical for our everyday lives. To do so, sometimes we need to step away from the hard numbers and apply quick and convenient methods that we can use anywhere and everywhere. That's why we measure our food using our own built-in portioning tools – our hands!
This proven method has been effectively applied in many nutrition programs for good reason—because it works. See the hand portion chart on the following page to start using this simple, effective method.

As long as you eat the approved foods in the portions that are right for you, the sky's the limit. Bon appétit!

HOW MUCH CAN I EAT?

For weight loss, not only is it essential to eat the right foods, but also that you eat the right amount of food. Your own hands provide one of the quickest and most convenient ways to portion your foods. Follow these simple guidelines to find portions that are appropriate for you.

Protein   Your portion of protein should be approximately the size and thickness of the palm of your hand.

Carbs   Your portion of carbs should be approximately the size of a clenched fist.

Fats   Your portion of fats should be approximately the size of your thumb from the base to the tip.

Veggies   Your portion of veggies should be approximately the size of two clenched fists. However, you can eat as many veggies as you like!

Flavorings   Your portion of flavorings should be no larger than the size of two fingers. That's all you'll need, and it keeps your calories under control!

Although using hand portions are fast and easy, they are not completely precise. If you want to determine the exact amount of calories you are consuming daily, use the 100-calorie portion chart that follows, which lists each of the acceptable foods in 100-calorie portions. In my experience, women who consume between 1,200 and 1,500 calories daily, and men who consume between 1,500 and 2,000 calories daily experience the most dramatic results. Taking these calorie estimates into consideration, you may adjust your hand portions if necessary to ensure you're eating portions that will help you reach your goals the fastest.

	Food	Women	Men
Protein	Powdered Protein	1 scoop	2 scoops
Carbs	Bread	1 slice	2 slices
	Corn Tortillas	2 tortillas	3 tortillas
	Brown Rice Tortillas	1 tortilla	2 tortillas
	Ezekiel Tortillas	1 tortilla	2 tortillas
	Whole Grain English Muffin	1/2 muffin	1 muffin

Sample Carb Cycle Week Calories from Sunday to Sunday

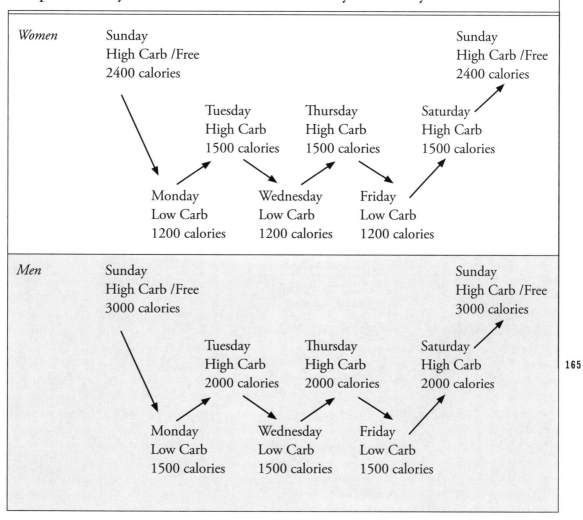

Women

Sunday
High Carb /Free
2400 calories

Tuesday
High Carb
1500 calories

Thursday
High Carb
1500 calories

Saturday
High Carb
1500 calories

Sunday
High Carb /Free
2400 calories

Monday
Low Carb
1200 calories

Wednesday
Low Carb
1200 calories

Friday
Low Carb
1200 calories

Men

Sunday
High Carb /Free
3000 calories

Tuesday
High Carb
2000 calories

Thursday
High Carb
2000 calories

Saturday
High Carb
2000 calories

Sunday
High Carb /Free
3000 calories

Monday
Low Carb
1500 calories

Wednesday
Low Carb
1500 calories

Friday
Low Carb
1500 calories

MEASURING UP

I know, I know—pulling out the measuring tools can be a pain in the butt. Although measuring your portions only takes a few extra seconds, it feels like a monumental task. But it's SO necessary. Don't you want to know if you're eating exactly the right portions to achieve the body you've always dreamed of?

Portion distortion is without a doubt one of the biggest nutritional problems we have in America. That's why I've calculated your portions for you on the 100-calorie chart. Measure them out for just a few days, and you'll know and understand your portions for life. You'll be able to eyeball something close to a proper portion from then on. If your weight loss begins to plateau, however, pull out those measuring tools again to make sure you're on track. . . . Sometimes your portions can creep back up!

TOOLS FOR **TRANSFORMATION**

One thing is certain: We love convenience. When it comes to food preparation, we want it fast, easy, and fun. Having the right gear on hand makes it easier to prepare your Carb-Cycle Solution meals. A few kitchen tools make food prep simple and convenient, allowing you to spend just minutes a day in the kitchen. What's also great is that these are one-time purchases, and you'll have these things for life. I don't require you to buy these tools, but I definitely recommend it!

I've found several items especially useful:
George Foreman grill
Rice cooker
Veggie steamer
Blender
Toaster oven
Shaker bottle (with blender ball)
Tupperware®-type containers
Kitchen scale
Measuring cups & spoons

	Approximately 100 Calories		Approximately 100 Calories
PROTEIN		Tofu	4 oz
Powdered		Tempeh	2 oz
Whey, Egg, Soy, Rice, Hemp Powdered Protein	1 scoop	Texturized Vegetable Protein	2 oz
Dairy		**CARBS**	
Egg Whites	4 whites	*Cereal*	
Egg Substitutes	1 cup	Steel Cut Oatmeal (cooked)	3/4 cup
Nonfat Plain Greek Yogurt	1 cup	Old Fashioned Oatmeal (cooked)	3/4 cup
Cottage Cheese	1 cup	Low-Fat Granola	1/2 cup
		Fiber One	3/4 cup
Poultry		All Bran	1/2 cup
Foster Farms Chicken Breast	3.5 oz	Kashi Go Lean	1/2 cup
Foster Farms Chicken Thighs	3 oz	Kashi Heart to Heart	3/4 cup
Turkey Breast (NOT DELI)	2.5 oz	Kashi Good Friends Cereal	1/2 cup
Lean Ground Meats		*Root Vegetables*	
Lean Ground Chicken Breast	2 oz	Sweet Potatoes / Yams	1/2 cup
Lean Ground Turkey	3 oz	Potatoes (Russet/Red/Gold)	3/4 cup
Low Sodium Deli Turkey	3.5 oz		
Ostrich / Duck Breast	2 oz	*Legumes*	
		Beans & Lentils (boiled or LOW SODIUM CANNED)	1/2 cup
Beef		Lentils (boiled or LOW SODIUM CANNED)	1/2 cup
Flank Steak	2 oz		
Round Steak	2 oz		
Cube Steak	2.5 oz	*Starchy Veggies*	
Ground Buffalo	1.5 oz	Peas	1 cup
Venison /Elk	2 oz	Corn	2/3 cup
		Carrots	2 cups
Seafood			
Tuna (canned)	3 oz	*Grains*	
Tuna (fillet)	3 oz	Long Grain Brown Rice	1/2 cup
Salmon (canned)	3.5 oz	Wild Rice	1/2 cup
Salmon (fillet)	2 oz	Barley	1/2 cup
Whitefish: Snapper/Halibut/ Cod/Trout/Catfish/Tilapia	2 oz	Amaranth	1/2 cup
		Couscous	1/2 cup
Shellfish: Scallops/Crab/ Lobster/Shrimp	4 oz	Quinoa	1/2 cup
		Buckwheat	1/2 cup

100-Calorie PORTION LIST

	Approximately 100 Calories		Approximately 100 Calories
Pasta		Cabbage	unlimited
Whole grain pasta	1/2 cup	Cucumber	unlimited
Brown Rice Pasta	1/2 cup	Sprouts	unlimited
		Squash	unlimited
Breads		Peppers	unlimited
Whole grain bread	1 slice	Parsley	unlimited
Ezekiel Breads	1 slice	Onions	unlimited
Ezekiel English Muffin	1/2 muffin	Collard Greens	unlimited
Ezekiel Tortillas	3/4 tortilla		
Brown Rice tortillas	1 tortilla	**FATS**	**70-100 Calories**
Corn Tortillas	1 1/2	Avocado	1/3 cup
tortillas		Pecans (raw, chopped)	1 1/2 Tbsp
		Almonds (raw, whole)	1 1/2 Tbsp
FRUIT		Walnuts (raw, chopped)	1 1/2 Tbsp
Berries	1 1/2 cups	Sunflower Seeds	1 1/2 Tbsp
Apples	1 1/2	Soy Nuts (roasted,	
Pears	1 pear	lightly salted)	3 Tbsp
Grapes	1 1/2 cups	Olives (large)	10.0
Orange / Tangerine	1.0	Egg Yolk	2.0
Peach /Nectarine	2.0	Creamy Dressing (Regular)	1 Tbsp
Plums	3.5	Creamy Dressing (Low-Fat)	2 Tbsp
Apricots	6.0	Heavy Whipping Cream	2 Tbsp
Kiwi	4.0	Mayonnaise, Regular	2 Tbsp
Melons	2.0	Cheese, Regular (1oz=1 slice)	1 oz
Banana	1.0	Cheese, Low-Fat (1oz=1 slice)	2 oz
Pineapple	1 1/3 cup		
		LIQUID FATS	
VEGGIES		Olive Oil	1 Tbsp
Spinach	unlimited	Flaxseed Oil	1 Tbsp
Lettuce	unlimited	Fish Oil	1 Tbsp
Eggplant	unlimited	Balsamic Vinaigrette	2 Tbsp
Tomatoes	unlimited	Almond Butter (with salt)	1 Tbsp
Mixed Greens	unlimited	Peanut Butter (with salt)	1 Tbsp
Broccoli	unlimited		
Asparagus	unlimited		
Cauliflower	unlimited		
Celery	unlimited		
Mushrooms	unlimited		
Green Beans	unlimited		
Zucchini	unlimited		

	Approximately 100 Calories		Approximately 100 Calories
FLAVORINGS	**30-50 Calories**	Lemon Juice	3 oz
Salsa (Newman's Own		Low-Fat Italian Dressing	
All-Natural)	1/2 cup	(Newman's Own LITE)	2 Tbsp
Tabasco	3 tsp	Fat-Free French Dressing	2 Tbsp
Marinara Sauce		Fat-Free Balsamic Vinaigrette	2 Tbsp
(Newman's Own)	1/2 cup	Fat-Free Mayo / Low-Fat Mayo	2 Tbsp
Chili Sauce	2 Tbsp	Butter Spray	5 sprays
Chili Paste	2 Tbsp	Mustard	3 tsp
Tomato Sauce	1/2 cup	Low Sodium Soy Sauce	3 tsp
Tomato Paste	3 Tbsp		
Hummus	2 Tbsp	Unsweetened Almond Milk	1 cup
Balsamic Vinegar	2 Tbsp	Low Sodium Chicken Broth	1 cup
Lime Juice	3 oz		

BUILDING A MEAL

Each of the dishes in the recipes section represents a properly portioned meal. If you're creating your own recipes, it's especially important to refer to the hand portions or 100-calorie portion chart to determine how much of each ingredient you can use to build each meal. When you invent your own dishes, it's also key to stick with the approved Carb-Cycle Solution foods. (If you deviate from the list, count non- approved items as cheat foods, and eat them only once every other day on your high-carb days OR as much as you want on your free day.)

Here's how to combine healthy portions of healthy ingredients into a healthy meal:

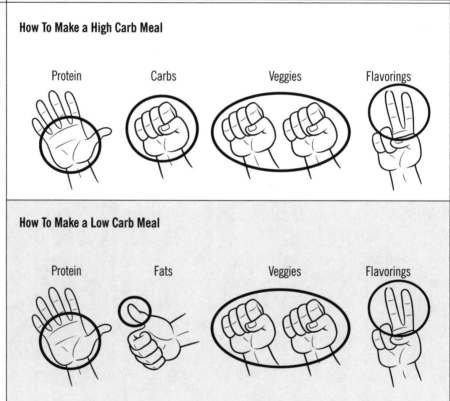

How To Make A **CARB-CYCLE MEAL**

How To Make a High Carb Meal

Protein   Carbs   Veggies   Flavorings

How To Make a Low Carb Meal

Protein   Fats   Veggies   Flavorings

INGREDIENTS	HIGH-CARB MEALS	LOW-CARB MEALS
Proteins	1 portion	1 portion
Carbohydrates	1 portion	None
Vegetables	Unlimited (except for root and starchy veggies in the carbohydrate category—they count as carbs)	Unlimited (except for root and starchy veggies in the carbohydrate category—they count as carbs)
Fats	None	1 portion
Flavorings	1 portion, plus unlimited herbs, spices, seasonings, and non-sugar sweeteners	1 portion, plus unlimited herbs, spices, seasonings, and non-sugar sweeteners

THE CARB-CYCLE SOLUTION RECIPES

Here they are—the recipes that are going to help you lose weight! These are so quick and easy that you'll have no excuse not to eat right. Each simple 200 to 300 calorie recipe makes up an entire meal. These recipes are scaled to general women's portions, so be sure to increase the portion size if necessary. But add as many servings as you like from the "Unlimited Vegetables" category in the Master Portion List. For extra-speedy meal tips, see the "Quick and Easy On-the-Go Foods" section in Chapter 9.

Be careful to eat high-carb dishes on high-carb days and low-carb dishes on low- carb days. The only exception is breakfast, which is always a high carb meal to start the day off right!

Note: You may season any of the recipes with salt and pepper to taste.

BREAKFAST, ANY DAY

FRUIT SMOOTHIE

Protein	1 scoop	Vanilla or Chocolate Protein Powder
Carb	1 cup	Banana or Berries
Drink	½ cup	Unsweetened Almond Milk

Directions

1 Blend together almond milk, 1 cup water, and protein powder.

2 Blend in banana or berries.

3 Blend with ice for desired thickness and enjoy!

BREAKFAST SANDWICH OR BREAKFAST TACOS

Protein	4	Egg Whites/Substitutes
Carb	½ 2	Whole-Grain or Ezekiel English Muffin OR Corn Tortillas
Veggie	3 slices	Tomato
Flavor	1 dash	Mrs. Dash®
	3 Tbsp	Salsa

Directions

1 Cook and stir egg whites in a skillet over medium heat until scrambled and done to your liking. Sprinkle with Mrs. Dash®.

2 Place scrambled egg whites on toasted English muffin or tortillas.

3 Add tomato and enjoy!

BREAKFAST, ANY DAY

POWER CRUNCH CEREAL

Protein	1 scoop	Vanilla Protein Powder
Carb	½ cup	Low-Fat Granola OR
	½ cup	All Bran OR
	¾ cup	Fiber One®
Drink	½ cup	Unsweetened Almond Milk
Flavor	to taste	Stevia
	to taste	Cinnamon

Directions

1 Blend almond milk and 1 cup water with protein powder, and add cinnamon and stevia to desired sweetness.

2 Pour over cereal and enjoy!

GREEK YOGURT AND BANANAS

Protein	1 cup	Nonfat Plain Greek Yogurt
Carb	1	Banana
Veggie	2 stalks	Celery
Flavor	1 dash	Stevia (optional)

Directions

1 Blend stevia with yogurt to desired sweetness.

2 Chop banana and mix into yogurt.

3 Enjoy with celery sticks on the side!

HIGH-CARB DAY: SNACKS, LUNCH, & DINNER

PROTEIN OATMEAL

Protein	1 scoop	Vanilla Protein Powder
Carb	¾ cup	Cooked Steel-Cut Oatmeal
Drink	½ cup	Unsweetened Almond Milk
Flavor	to taste	Stevia
	to taste	Cinnamon

Directions

1 Blend almond milk and 1 cup water with protein powder, cinnamon, and stevia to desired sweetness.

2 According to instructions on package, bring water to a boil, and stir in oatmeal. Let simmer per instructions; stir occasionally.

3 Pour protein shake over the oatmeal, mix, and enjoy!

CHOCOLATE-OATMEAL POWER SHAKE

Protein	1 scoop	Chocolate Protein Powder
Carb	¾ cup	Old-Fashioned Oatmeal (cooked)
Drink	½ cup	Unsweetened Almond Milk

Directions

1 Blend almond milk with 1 cup water and protein powder.

2 Blend in oatmeal for a hearty shake.

3 Blend with ice for desired thickness and enjoy!

HIGH-CARB DAY: SNACKS, LUNCH, & DINNER

YOGURT CRUNCH

Protein	1 cup	Nonfat Greek Yogurt
Carb	½ cup	Low-Fat Granola
Flavor	1 dash	Stevia

Directions

1 Blend yogurt and stevia to desired sweetness.

2 Mix in granola and enjoy!

TURKEY & VEGGIE MEDLEY

Protein	3 oz	Cooked Extra-Lean Ground Turkey
Carb	½ cup mixed	Cooked Peas and Corn
	⅓ cup	Cooked Long-Grain Brown Rice
Flavor	5 Sprays to taste	Spray Butter Herb & Garlic Mrs. Dash®

Directions

1 Lightly sprinkle turkey with Mrs. Dash®, then spray lightly with spray butter.

2 Mix turkey with rice, peas, and corn.

3 Heat on stovetop or in microwave.

HIGH-CARB DAY: SNACKS, LUNCH, & DINNER

CHICKEN STIR-FRY

Protein	3 ½ oz	Cooked, Sliced Chicken Breast
Carb	½ cup	Cooked Long-Grain Brown Rice
Veggie	3 cups mixed	Steamed Broccoli, Mushrooms, Green Beans, and Water Chestnuts
Flavor	1 tsp	Low-Sodium Soy Sauce
	to taste	Mrs. Dash®

Directions

1 Spray non-stick cooking spray in a skillet, and heat chicken and veggies.
2 Sprinkle with Mrs. Dash®, and drizzle with soy sauce.
3 Serve with rice and enjoy!

CHICKEN TOSTADAS

Protein	3 ½ oz	Cooked Chicken Breast
Carb	1	Corn Tortillas
	⅓ cup	Boiled or Canned Black Beans
Veggie	2 cups mixed	Chopped Onions and Peppers
	1 cup	Chopped Iceberg Lettuce
Flavor	3 Tbsp	Salsa

Directions

1 Lightly spray a large skillet with non-stick cooking spray, and set stove to medium heat. Sauté onions, peppers, and chicken for 5 minutes.
2 Mix in beans and heat.
3 Remove from heat, and mix with lettuce and salsa.
4 Tear tortillas into 1-inch pieces, and sprinkle over the top.
5 (Optional: Heat on stovetop or in microwave.) Enjoy!

HIGH-CARB DAY: SNACKS, LUNCH, & DINNER

CHICKEN MARINARA PASTA

Protein	3 ½ oz	Cooked, Chopped Chicken Breast
Carb	½ cup	Cooked Brown-Rice Pasta
Veggie	½ cup	Sautéed Sliced Mushrooms
	1 cup	Steamed Broccoli
Flavor	1 Tbsp	Minced Garlic
	3 Tbsp	Marinara Sauce

Directions

1 Mix together chicken breast, garlic, mushrooms, broccoli, and marinara sauce.

2 Toss with pasta.

3 Heat on stovetop or in microwave and enjoy!

STEAK 'N' POTATOES

Protein	2 oz	Thinly Sliced Cooked Flank Steak
Carb	1 small	Yam or Gold Potato
Veggie	½ cup	Chopped Onions
	½ cup	Sliced Mushrooms
Flavor	to taste	Mrs. Dash®
	5 Sprays	Spray Butter
	1 tsp	Cinnamon for Yam OR
	3 Tbsp	Marinara Sauce for Potato

Directions

1 Bake yam or potato in microwave or conventional oven.

2 Spray skillet with non-stick cooking spray. Lightly sauté the onions and mushrooms for about 5 minutes. Season with Mrs. Dash®.

3 Add steak and heat.

4 Split open yam or potato. Spray with butter spray. Sprinkle yam with cinnamon or top potato with marinara sauce.

5 Place steak mixture and yam or potato on a dinner plate. Enjoy!

HIGH-CARB DAY: SNACKS, LUNCH, & DINNER

MEDITERRANEAN TURKEY

Protein	3 oz	Cooked Extra-Lean Ground Turkey
Carb	½ cup	Cooked Long-Grain Brown Rice
Veggie	1 cup	Steamed Broccoli
	1 cup	Steamed Cauliflower
Flavor	1 Tbsp	Hummus
	to taste	Garlic & Herb Mrs. Dash®

Directions

1 Mix together turkey, broccoli, and cauliflower. Sprinkle with Mrs. Dash®.

2 Mix in rice.

3 Top with hummus.

4 (Optional: Heat on stovetop or in microwave.) Enjoy!

GRILLED SHRIMP PASTA

Protein	4 oz	Grilled Shrimp
Carb	½ cup	Cooked Brown-Rice Pasta
Veggie	1 cup	Steamed Broccoli
Flavor	to taste	Garlic & Herb Mrs. Dash®
	5 sprays	Spray Butter

Directions

1 Toss shrimp and broccoli with Mrs. Dash®.

2 Mix in pasta.

3 Spray lightly with spray butter and enjoy!

HIGH-CARB DAY: SNACKS, LUNCH, & DINNER

SPICY TEX-MEX TURKEY

Protein	3 oz	Cooked Extra-Lean Ground Turkey
Carb	⅓ cup	Cooked Corn
	⅓ cup	Boiled or Canned Black Beans
Veggie	1 cup	Chopped Red Bell Peppers
Flavor	2 tsp	Tabasco Sauce
	3 Tbsp	Salsa

Directions

1   Mix together turkey, corn, beans, and peppers.

2   Stir in salsa and Tabasco to spice things up!

3   (Optional: Heat on stovetop or in microwave.) Enjoy!

TUNA SANDWICH

Protein	3 oz	Canned Tuna
Carb	1 slice	Ezekiel® Bread
Veggie	2 leaves	Iceberg Lettuce
	2 slices	Tomato
	¼ sliced	Onion
Flavor	2 Tbsp	Fat-Free Mayonnaise
	to taste	Black Pepper

Directions

1   Mix the tuna with mayonnaise and pepper.

2   Spread the tuna salad on one slice of bread.

3   Stack on the lettuce, tomatoes, and onions.

4   Eat cold or toast the sandwich and enjoy!

LOW-CARB DAY: SNACKS, LUNCH, & DINNER

COTTAGE CHEESE ON-THE-BORDER

Protein	1 cup	Nonfat Cottage Cheese
Veggie	½ cup	Chopped Tomato
Fat	⅓	Avocado, Sliced
Flavor	3 Tbsp	Salsa

Directions

1 Blend cottage cheese and salsa.

2 Mix in tomato.

3 Serve avocado on the side or mixed in. Enjoy!

TURKEY-LETTUCE TACO MIX

Protein	3 oz	Cooked Extra-Lean Ground Turkey
Veggie	⅔ cup	Chopped Iceberg Lettuce
Fat	2 oz	Grated Low-Fat Cheddar Cheese
Flavor	3 Tbsp	Salsa

Directions

1 Toss turkey with salsa and lettuce.

2 Sprinkle on cheese.

3 (Optional: Heat on stovetop or in microwave.) Enjoy!

LOW-CARB DAY: SNACKS, LUNCH, & DINNER

CHOCOLATE-PEANUT BUTTER SHAKE

Protein	1 scoop	Chocolate Protein Powder
Fat	1 Tbsp	Natural Peanut Butter
Drink	½ cup	Unsweetened Almond Milk

Directions
1 Blend almond milk with 1 cup water and protein powder.
2 Blend in peanut butter.
3 Blend with ice for desired thickness and enjoy!

ASIAN WRAPS

Protein	3 oz	Cooked Extra-Lean Ground Chicken Breast or Ground Turkey
Veggie	¼ cup each	Chopped Water Chestnuts, Tomato, Onions
	1 leaf	Iceberg Lettuce
Fat	⅓	Avocado, Sliced
Flavor	1 Tbsp	Low-Sodium Soy Sauce

Directions
1 Arrange chicken or turkey, water chestnuts, tomatoes, and onions on lettuce leaf.
2 Drizzle with soy sauce.
3 Place avocado on top.
4 Wrap and enjoy!

LOW-CARB DAY: SNACKS, LUNCH, & DINNER

CHICKEN COBB SALAD

Protein	2	Chopped Hard-Boiled Egg Whites
	2 oz	Chopped Chicken Breast
Veggie	3 cups mixed	Chopped Tomato, Cucumber, Iceberg Lettuce
Fat	1 Tbsp	Blue Cheese Crumbles
	¼	Avocado, Chopped
Flavor	2 Tbsp	Fat-Free Balsamic Vinaigrette

Directions

1 Combine chicken, egg whites, lettuce, tomatoes, cucumbers, and avocado.

2 Sprinkle cheese on top. Drizzle with vinaigrette.

3 Toss and enjoy!

CHICKEN-VEGGIE PARMESAN

Protein	4 oz	Cooked, Sliced Chicken Breast
Veggie	3 cups mixed	Steamed, Chopped Zucchini, Spinach, Mushrooms
Fat	2 oz	Low-Fat Parmesan Cheese
Flavor	3 Tbsp	Marinara Sauce
	to taste	Herb & Garlic Mrs. Dash®

Directions

1 Mix chicken with zucchini, mushrooms, and spinach. Heat on stovetop or in microwave.

2 Sprinkle with Mrs. Dash®, and pour on marinara.

3 Melt cheese over the top in microwave and enjoy!

LOW-CARB DAY: SNACKS, LUNCH, & DINNER

GARLIC-HERB SALMON SALAD

Protein	2 oz	Grilled Salmon
Veggie	2 cups	Uncooked Spinach
Fat	2 Tbsp	Balsamic Vinaigrette
Flavor	1 Tbsp	Lemon Juice
	1 dash	Garlic & Herb Mrs. Dash®
	1 Tbsp	Sautéed Minced Garlic

Directions

1 Spread sautéed garlic on salmon and sprinkle with Mrs. Dash®.

2 Lay fish on a bed of spinach and sprinkle with lemon juice.

3 Drizzle vinaigrette over the top.

4 (Optional: Heat in microwave.) Enjoy!

LEMON-PEPPER TILAPIA

Protein	3 oz	Baked Tilapia Fillet
Veggie	½ cup	Steamed Sliced Mushrooms
	10 stalks	Steamed Asparagus
Fat	1 Tbsp	Sliced Almonds
Flavor	1 Tbsp	Lemon Juice
	1 dash	Lemon-Pepper Mrs. Dash®
	5 sprays	Spray Butter

Directions

1 Arrange asparagus on a plate and top with mushrooms.

2 Lay the tilapia on top. Sprinkle with lemon juice and Mrs. Dash®.

3 Spray fish lightly with spray butter, and sprinkle almonds over the top.

4 (Optional: Heat on stovetop or in microwave.) Enjoy!

LOW-CARB DAY: SNACKS, LUNCH, & DINNER

SUNSHINE OMELET

Protein	4	Egg Whites
Veggie	½ cup	Sliced Mushrooms
	½ cup	Chopped Onions
	½ cup	Chopped Tomatoes
Fat	2 oz	Grated Low-Fat Mozzarella Cheese
Flavor	to taste	Mrs. Dash®

Directions

1 Spray a skillet with non-stick spray and heat. Blend egg whites, and pour into hot pan.

2 When whites start to cook, toss on onions, mushrooms, and tomatoes.

3 Sprinkle with Mrs. Dash®, and top with cheese.

4 Wait for whites to cook through, fold omelet in half and enjoy!

ITALIAN TURKEY

Protein	3 oz	Cooked Extra-Lean Ground Turkey
Veggie	1	Chopped Bell Pepper
	1 cup	Sliced Mushrooms
	1 cup	Spinach
Fat	2 oz	Grated Low-Fat Mozzarella Cheese
Flavor	3 Tbsp	Marinara Sauce

Directions

1 Sauté turkey with pepper, mushrooms, and spinach.

2 Stir in marinara sauce and heat.

3 Sprinkle cheese on top.

4 (Optional: Heat on stovetop or in microwave.) Enjoy!

LOW-CARB DAY: SNACKS, LUNCH, & DINNER

STEAK 'N' GREEN BEANS

Protein	2 oz	Cooked, Sliced Flank Steak
Veggie	2 cups	Steamed Green Beans
Fat	2 Tbsp	Sliced Almonds
Flavor	5 sprays	Spray Butter
	to taste	Mrs. Dash®

Directions

1 Toss steak with beans. Season with Mrs. Dash® and spray butter.

2 Sprinkle almonds over the top.

3 (Optional: Heat on stovetop or in microwave.) Enjoy!

TUNA-SPINACH SALAD

Protein	3 oz	Canned Tuna
Veggie	3 cups	Uncooked Spinach
Fat	1 Tbsp	Low-Fat Mayonnaise
	1 Tbsp	Balsamic Vinaigrette
Flavor	to taste	Lemon-Pepper Mrs. Dash®

Directions

1 Mix tuna with mayonnaise and Mrs. Dash®.

2 Spoon onto a bed of spinach.

3 Drizzle with vinaigrette and enjoy!

APPENDIX A - 12 WEEKS OF SAMPLE CARB-CYCLE SCHEDULES

WEEK 1

Carb Cycle Week Sample Schedule	Monday	Tuesday	Wednesday	Thursday	Friday	Saturday	Sunday
6am wake up	Sprint Shaper _____rounds in 10 minutes		Endurance Shaper _____reps push ups _____reps sit ups _____reps squats		Size and Shape Shaper _____rounds in 5 minutes _____rounds in 5 minutes		Free Day
within 30 minutes of waking	High Carb Breakfast	High Carb Breakfast	High Carb Breakfast	High Carb Breakfast	High Carb Breakfast	High Carb Breakfast	High Carb Breakfast
9am	Low Carb Snack	High Carb Snack	Low Carb Snack	High Carb Snack	Low Carb Snack	High Carb Snack	High Carb Snack
12pm	Low Carb Lunch	High Carb Lunch	Low Carb Lunch	High Carb Lunch	Low Carb Lunch	High Carb Lunch	High Carb Lunch
	I completed __ Shredders Goal: 5 Shredders	I completed __ Shredders Goal: 5 Shredders	I completed __ Shredders Goal: 5 Shredders	I completed __ Shredders Goal: 5 Shredders	I completed __ Shredders Goal: 5 Shredders	I completed __ Shredders Goal: 5 Shredders	
3pm	Low Carb Snack	High Carb Snack	Low Carb Snack	High Carb Snack	Low Carb Snack	High Carb Snack	High Carb Snack
6pm	Low Carb Dinner	High Carb Dinner	Low Carb Dinner	High Carb Dinner	Low Carb Dinner	High Carb Dinner	High Carb Dinner

*The clock starts as soon as you wake up, and each meal should be spaced approximately three hours apart.

Note: Shredders can be completed at any time during the day.

APPENDIX A - 12 WEEKS OF SAMPLE CARB-CYCLE SCHEDULES

Carb Cycle Week Sample Schedule	Monday	Tuesday	Wednesday	Thursday	Friday	Saturday	Sunday
6am wake up	Sprint Shaper _____rounds in 10 minutes		Endurance Shaper _____reps push ups _____reps sit ups _____reps squats		Size and Shape Shaper _____rounds in 5 minutes _____rounds in 5 minutes		Free Day
within 30 minutes of waking	High Carb Breakfast	High Carb Breakfast	High Carb Breakfast	High Carb Breakfast	High Carb Breakfast	High Carb Breakfast	High Carb Breakfast
9am	Low Carb Snack	High Carb Snack	Low Carb Snack	High Carb Snack	Low Carb Snack	High Carb Snack	High Carb Snack
12pm	Low Carb Lunch I completed ___ Shredders Goal: 5 Shredders	High Carb Lunch I completed ___ Shredders Goal: 5 Shredders	Low Carb Lunch I completed ___ Shredders Goal: 5 Shredders	High Carb Lunch I completed ___ Shredders Goal: 5 Shredders	Low Carb Lunch I completed ___ Shredders Goal: 5 Shredders	High Carb Lunch I completed ___ Shredders Goal: 5 Shredders	High Carb Lunch
3pm	Low Carb Snack	High Carb Snack	Low Carb Snack	High Carb Snack	Low Carb Snack	High Carb Snack	High Carb Snack
6pm	Low Carb Dinner	High Carb Dinner	Low Carb Dinner	High Carb Dinner	Low Carb Dinner	High Carb Dinner	High Carb Dinner

*The clock starts as soon as you wake up, and each meal should be spaced approximately three hours apart.

Note: Shredders can be completed at any time during the day.

APPENDIX A - 12 WEEKS OF SAMPLE CARB-CYCLE SCHEDULES

WEEK 3

Carb Cycle Week Sample Schedule	Monday	Tuesday	Wednesday	Thursday	Friday	Saturday	Sunday
6am wake up	Sprint Shaper _____rounds in 10 minutes		Endurance Shaper _____reps push ups _____reps sit ups _____reps squats		Size and Shape Shaper _____rounds in 5 minutes _____rounds in 5 minutes		Free Day
within 30 minutes of waking	High Carb Breakfast	High Carb Breakfast	High Carb Breakfast	High Carb Breakfast	High Carb Breakfast	High Carb Breakfast	High Carb Breakfast
9am	Low Carb Snack	High Carb Snack	Low Carb Snack	High Carb Snack	Low Carb Snack	High Carb Snack	High Carb Snack
12pm	Low Carb Lunch I completed __ Shredders Goal: 6 Shredders	High Carb Lunch I completed __ Shredders Goal: 6 Shredders	Low Carb Lunch I completed __ Shredders Goal: 6 Shredders	High Carb Lunch I completed __ Shredders Goal: 6 Shredders	Low Carb Lunch I completed __ Shredders Goal: 6 Shredders	High Carb Lunch I completed __ Shredders Goal: 6 Shredders	High Carb Lunch
3pm	Low Carb Snack	High Carb Snack	Low Carb Snack	High Carb Snack	Low Carb Snack	High Carb Snack	High Carb Snack
6pm	Low Carb Dinner	High Carb Dinner	Low Carb Dinner	High Carb Dinner	Low Carb Dinner	High Carb Dinner	High Carb Dinner

*The clock starts as soon as you wake up, and each meal should be spaced approximately three hours apart.

Note: Shredders can be completed at any time during the day.

APPENDIX A - 12 WEEKS OF SAMPLE CARB-CYCLE SCHEDULES

Slingshot Week Sample Schedule	Monday	Tuesday	Wednesday	Thursday	Friday	Saturday	Sunday
6am wake up	Sprint Shaper _____rounds in 10 minutes		Endurance Shaper _____reps push ups _____reps sit ups _____reps squats		Size and Shape Shaper _____rounds in 5 minutes _____rounds in 5 minutes		Free Day
within 30 minutes of waking	High Carb Breakfast	High Carb Breakfast	High Carb Breakfast	High Carb Breakfast	High Carb Breakfast	High Carb Breakfast	High Carb Breakfast
9am	High Carb Snack	High Carb Snack	High Carb Snack	High Carb Snack	High Carb Snack	High Carb Snack	High Carb Snack
12pm	High Carb Lunch I completed __ Shredders Goal: 6 Shredders	High Carb Lunch I completed __ Shredders Goal: 6 Shredders	High Carb Lunch I completed __ Shredders Goal: 6 Shredders	High Carb Lunch I completed __ Shredders Goal: 6 Shredders	High Carb Lunch I completed __ Shredders Goal: 6 Shredders	High Carb Lunch I completed __ Shredders Goal: 6 Shredders	High Carb Lunch
3pm	High Carb Snack	High Carb Snack	High Carb Snack	High Carb Snack	High Carb Snack	High Carb Snack	High Carb Snack
6pm	High Carb Dinner	High Carb Dinner	High Carb Dinner	High Carb Dinner	High Carb Dinner	High Carb Dinner	High Carb Dinner

*The clock starts as soon as you wake up, and each meal should be spaced approximately three hours apart.

Note: Shredders can be completed at any time during the day.

APPENDIX A - 12 WEEKS OF SAMPLE CARB-CYCLE SCHEDULES

WEEK 5

Carb Cycle Week Sample Schedule	Monday	Tuesday	Wednesday	Thursday	Friday	Saturday	Sunday
6am wake up	Sprint Shaper _____rounds in 10 minutes		Endurance Shaper _____reps push ups _____reps sit ups _____reps squats		Size and Shape Shaper _____rounds in 5 minutes _____rounds in 5 minutes		Free Day
within 30 minutes of waking	High Carb Breakfast	High Carb Breakfast	High Carb Breakfast	High Carb Breakfast	High Carb Breakfast	High Carb Breakfast	High Carb Breakfast
9am	Low Carb Snack	High Carb Snack	Low Carb Snack	High Carb Snack	Low Carb Snack	High Carb Snack	High Carb Snack
12pm	Low Carb Lunch I completed __ Shredders Goal: 7 Shredders	High Carb Lunch I completed __ Shredders Goal: 7 Shredders	Low Carb Lunch I completed __ Shredders Goal: 7 Shredders	High Carb Lunch I completed __ Shredders Goal: 7 Shredders	Low Carb Lunch I completed __ Shredders Goal: 7 Shredders	High Carb Lunch I completed __ Shredders Goal: 7 Shredders	High Carb Lunch
3pm	Low Carb Snack	High Carb Snack	Low Carb Snack	High Carb Snack	Low Carb Snack	High Carb Snack	High Carb Snack
6pm	Low Carb Dinner	High Carb Dinner	Low Carb Dinner	High Carb Dinner	Low Carb Dinner	High Carb Dinner	High Carb Dinner

*The clock starts as soon as you wake up, and each meal should be spaced approximately three hours apart.

Note: Shredders can be completed at any time during the day.

APPENDIX A - 12 WEEKS OF SAMPLE CARB-CYCLE SCHEDULES

WEEK 6

Slingshot Week Sample Schedule	Monday	Tuesday	Wednesday	Thursday	Friday	Saturday	Sunday
6am wake up	Sprint Shaper _____rounds in 10 minutes		Endurance Shaper _____reps push ups _____reps sit ups _____reps squats		Size and Shape Shaper _____rounds in 5 minutes _____rounds in 5 minutes		Free Day
within 30 minutes of waking	High Carb Breakfast	High Carb Breakfast	High Carb Breakfast	High Carb Breakfast	High Carb Breakfast	High Carb Breakfast	High Carb Breakfast
9am	Low Carb Snack	High Carb Snack	Low Carb Snack	High Carb Snack	Low Carb Snack	High Carb Snack	High Carb Snack
12pm	Low Carb Lunch I completed ___ Shredders Goal: 7 Shredders	High Carb Lunch I completed ___ Shredders Goal: 7 Shredders	Low Carb Lunch I completed ___ Shredders Goal: 7 Shredders	High Carb Lunch I completed ___ Shredders Goal: 7 Shredders	Low Carb Lunch I completed ___ Shredders Goal: 7 Shredders	High Carb Lunch I completed ___ Shredders Goal: 7 Shredders	High Carb Lunch
3pm	Low Carb Snack	High Carb Snack	Low Carb Snack	High Carb Snack	Low Carb Snack	High Carb Snack	High Carb Snack
6pm	Low Carb Dinner	High Carb Dinner	Low Carb Dinner	High Carb Dinner	Low Carb Dinner	High Carb Dinner	High Carb Dinner

*The clock starts as soon as you wake up, and each meal should be spaced approximately three hours apart.

Note: Shredders can be completed at any time during the day.

APPENDIX A - 12 WEEKS OF SAMPLE CARB-CYCLE SCHEDULES

WEEK 7

Carb Cycle Week Sample Schedule	Monday	Tuesday	Wednesday	Thursday	Friday	Saturday	Sunday
6am wake up	Sprint Shaper _____rounds in 10 minutes		Endurance Shaper _____reps push ups _____reps sit ups _____reps squats		Size and Shape Shaper _____rounds in 5 minutes _____rounds in 5 minutes		Free Day
within 30 minutes of waking	High Carb Breakfast	High Carb Breakfast	High Carb Breakfast	High Carb Breakfast	High Carb Breakfast	High Carb Breakfast	High Carb Breakfast
9am	Low Carb Snack	High Carb Snack	Low Carb Snack	High Carb Snack	Low Carb Snack	High Carb Snack	High Carb Snack
12pm	Low Carb Lunch I completed __ Shredders Goal: 8 Shredders	High Carb Lunch I completed __ Shredders Goal: 8 Shredders	Low Carb Lunch I completed __ Shredders Goal: 8 Shredders	High Carb Lunch I completed __ Shredders Goal: 8 Shredders	Low Carb Lunch I completed __ Shredders Goal: 8 Shredders	High Carb Lunch I completed __ Shredders Goal: 8 Shredders	High Carb Lunch
3pm	Low Carb Snack	High Carb Snack	Low Carb Snack	High Carb Snack	Low Carb Snack	High Carb Snack	High Carb Snack
6pm	Low Carb Dinner	High Carb Dinner	Low Carb Dinner	High Carb Dinner	Low Carb Dinner	High Carb Dinner	High Carb Dinner

*The clock starts as soon as you wake up, and each meal should be spaced approximately three hours apart.

Note: Shredders can be completed at any time during the day.

APPENDIX A - 12 WEEKS OF SAMPLE CARB-CYCLE SCHEDULES

Slingshot Week Sample Schedule	Monday	Tuesday	Wednesday	Thursday	Friday	Saturday	Sunday
6am wake up	Sprint Shaper _____rounds in 10 minutes		Endurance Shaper _____reps push ups _____reps sit ups _____reps squats		Size and Shape Shaper _____rounds in 5 minutes _____rounds in 5 minutes		Free Day
within 30 minutes of waking	High Carb Breakfast	High Carb Breakfast	High Carb Breakfast	High Carb Breakfast	High Carb Breakfast	High Carb Breakfast	High Carb Breakfast
9am	High Carb Snack	High Carb Snack	High Carb Snack	High Carb Snack	High Carb Snack	High Carb Snack	High Carb Snack
12pm	High Carb Lunch	High Carb Lunch	High Carb Lunch	High Carb Lunch	High Carb Lunch	High Carb Lunch	High Carb Lunch
	I completed __ Shredders Goal: 8 Shredders	I completed __ Shredders Goal: 8 Shredders	I completed __ Shredders Goal: 8 Shredders	I completed __ Shredders Goal: 8 Shredders	I completed __ Shredders Goal: 8 Shredders	I completed __ Shredders Goal: 8 Shredders	
3pm	High Carb Snack	High Carb Snack	High Carb Snack	High Carb Snack	High Carb Snack	High Carb Snack	High Carb Snack
6pm	High Carb Dinner	High Carb Dinner	High Carb Dinner	High Carb Dinner	High Carb Dinner	High Carb Dinner	High Carb Dinner

*The clock starts as soon as you wake up, and each meal should be spaced approximately three hours apart.

Note: Shredders can be completed at any time during the day.

APPENDIX A - 12 WEEKS OF SAMPLE CARB-CYCLE SCHEDULES

WEEK 9

Carb Cycle Week Sample Schedule	Monday	Tuesday	Wednesday	Thursday	Friday	Saturday	Sunday
6am wake up	Sprint Shaper _____rounds in 10 minutes		Endurance Shaper _____reps push ups _____reps sit ups _____reps squats		Size and Shape Shaper _____rounds in 5 minutes _____rounds in 5 minutes		Free Day
within 30 minutes of waking	High Carb Breakfast	High Carb Breakfast	High Carb Breakfast	High Carb Breakfast	High Carb Breakfast	High Carb Breakfast	High Carb Breakfast
9am	Low Carb Snack	High Carb Snack	Low Carb Snack	High Carb Snack	Low Carb Snack	High Carb Snack	High Carb Snack
12pm	Low Carb Lunch I completed ___ Shredders Goal: 9 Shredders	High Carb Lunch I completed ___ Shredders Goal: 9 Shredders	Low Carb Lunch I completed ___ Shredders Goal: 9 Shredders	High Carb Lunch I completed ___ Shredders Goal: 9 Shredders	Low Carb Lunch I completed ___ Shredders Goal: 9 Shredders	High Carb Lunch I completed ___ Shredders Goal: 9 Shredders	High Carb Lunch
3pm	Low Carb Snack	High Carb Snack	Low Carb Snack	High Carb Snack	Low Carb Snack	High Carb Snack	High Carb Snack
6pm	Low Carb Dinner	High Carb Dinner	Low Carb Dinner	High Carb Dinner	Low Carb Dinner	High Carb Dinner	High Carb Dinner

*The clock starts as soon as you wake up, and each meal should be spaced approximately three hours apart.

Note: Shredders can be completed at any time during the day.

APPENDIX A - 12 WEEKS OF SAMPLE CARB-CYCLE SCHEDULES

Slingshot Week Sample Schedule	Monday	Tuesday	Wednesday	Thursday	Friday	Saturday	Sunday
6am wake up	Sprint Shaper _____rounds in 10 minutes		Endurance Shaper _____reps push ups _____reps sit ups _____reps squats		Size and Shape Shaper _____rounds in 5 minutes _____rounds in 5 minutes		Free Day
within 30 minutes of waking	High Carb Breakfast	High Carb Breakfast	High Carb Breakfast	High Carb Breakfast	High Carb Breakfast	High Carb Breakfast	High Carb Breakfast
9am	Low Carb Snack	High Carb Snack	Low Carb Snack	High Carb Snack	Low Carb Snack	High Carb Snack	High Carb Snack
12pm	Low Carb Lunch I completed __ Shredders Goal: 9 Shredders	High Carb Lunch I completed __ Shredders Goal: 9 Shredders	Low Carb Lunch I completed __ Shredders Goal: 9 Shredders	High Carb Lunch I completed __ Shredders Goal: 9 Shredders	Low Carb Lunch I completed __ Shredders Goal: 9 Shredders	High Carb Lunch I completed __ Shredders Goal: 9 Shredders	High Carb Lunch
3pm	Low Carb Snack	High Carb Snack	Low Carb Snack	High Carb Snack	Low Carb Snack	High Carb Snack	High Carb Snack
6pm	Low Carb Dinner	High Carb Dinner	Low Carb Dinner	High Carb Dinner	Low Carb Dinner	High Carb Dinner	High Carb Dinner

*The clock starts as soon as you wake up, and each meal should be spaced approximately three hours apart.

Note: Shredders can be completed at any time during the day.

APPENDIX A - 12 WEEKS OF SAMPLE CARB-CYCLE SCHEDULES

WEEK 11

Carb Cycle Week Sample Schedule	Monday	Tuesday	Wednesday	Thursday	Friday	Saturday	Sunday
6am wake up	Sprint Shaper _____rounds in 10 minutes		Endurance Shaper _____reps push ups _____reps sit ups _____reps squats		Size and Shape Shaper _____rounds in 5 minutes _____rounds in 5 minutes		Free Day
within 30 minutes of waking	High Carb Breakfast	High Carb Breakfast	High Carb Breakfast	High Carb Breakfast	High Carb Breakfast	High Carb Breakfast	High Carb Breakfast
9am	Low Carb Snack	High Carb Snack	Low Carb Snack	High Carb Snack	Low Carb Snack	High Carb Snack	High Carb Snack
12pm	Low Carb Lunch I completed __ Shredders Goal: 10 Shredders	High Carb Lunch I completed __ Shredders Goal: 10 Shredders	Low Carb Lunch I completed __ Shredders Goal: 10 Shredders	High Carb Lunch I completed __ Shredders Goal: 10 Shredders	Low Carb Lunch I completed __ Shredders Goal: 10 Shredders	High Carb Lunch I completed __ Shredders Goal: 10 Shredders	High Carb Lunch
3pm	Low Carb Snack	High Carb Snack	Low Carb Snack	High Carb Snack	Low Carb Snack	High Carb Snack	High Carb Snack
6pm	Low Carb Dinner	High Carb Dinner	Low Carb Dinner	High Carb Dinner	Low Carb Dinner	High Carb Dinner	High Carb Dinner

*The clock starts as soon as you wake up, and each meal should be spaced approximately three hours apart.

Note: Shredders can be completed at any time during the day.

APPENDIX A - 12 WEEKS OF SAMPLE CARB-CYCLE SCHEDULES

Slingshot Week Sample Schedule	Monday	Tuesday	Wednesday	Thursday	Friday	Saturday	Sunday
6am wake up	Sprint Shaper _____rounds in 10 minutes		Endurance Shaper _____reps push ups _____reps sit ups _____reps squats		Size and Shape Shaper _____rounds in 5 minutes _____rounds in 5 minutes		Free Day
within 30 minutes of waking	High Carb Breakfast	High Carb Breakfast	High Carb Breakfast	High Carb Breakfast	High Carb Breakfast	High Carb Breakfast	High Carb Breakfast
9am	High Carb Snack	High Carb Snack	High Carb Snack	High Carb Snack	High Carb Snack	High Carb Snack	High Carb Snack
12pm	High Carb Lunch I completed ___ Shredders Goal: 10 Shredders	High Carb Lunch I completed ___ Shredders Goal: 10 Shredders	High Carb Lunch I completed ___ Shredders Goal: 10 Shredders	High Carb Lunch I completed ___ Shredders Goal: 10 Shredders	High Carb Lunch I completed ___ Shredders Goal: 10 Shredders	High Carb Lunch I completed ___ Shredders Goal: 10 Shredders	High Carb Lunch
3pm	High Carb Snack	High Carb Snack	High Carb Snack	High Carb Snack	High Carb Snack	High Carb Snack	High Carb Snack
6pm	High Carb Dinner	High Carb Dinner	High Carb Dinner	High Carb Dinner	High Carb Dinner	High Carb Dinner	High Carb Dinner

*The clock starts as soon as you wake up, and each meal should be spaced approximately three hours apart.

Note: Shredders can be completed at any time during the day.

APPENDIX B - BODY MASS INDEX TABLE 1

for BMI greater than 35, go to Table 2

To use the table, find the appropriate height in the left-hand column labeled Height. Move across to a given weight (in pounds). The number at the top of the column is the BMI at that height and weight. Pounds have been rounded off.

BMI	19	20	21	22	23	24	25	26	27	28	29	30	31	32	33	34	35
Height (inches)	Body Weight (pounds)																
58	91	96	100	105	110	115	119	124	129	134	138	143	148	153	158	162	167
59	94	99	104	109	114	119	124	128	133	138	143	148	153	158	163	168	173
60	97	102	107	112	118	123	128	133	138	143	148	153	158	163	168	174	179
61	100	106	111	116	122	127	132	137	143	148	153	158	164	169	174	180	185
62	104	109	115	120	126	131	136	142	147	153	158	164	169	175	180	186	191
63	107	113	118	124	130	135	141	146	152	158	163	169	175	180	186	191	197
64	110	116	122	128	134	140	145	151	157	163	169	174	180	186	192	197	204
65	114	120	126	132	138	144	150	156	162	168	174	180	186	192	198	204	210
66	118	124	130	136	142	148	155	161	167	173	179	186	192	198	204	210	216
67	121	127	134	140	146	153	159	166	172	178	185	191	198	204	211	217	223
68	125	131	138	144	151	158	164	171	177	184	190	197	203	210	216	223	230
69	128	135	142	149	155	162	169	176	182	189	196	203	209	216	223	230	236
70	132	139	146	153	160	167	174	181	188	195	202	209	216	222	229	236	243
71	136	143	150	157	165	172	179	186	193	200	208	215	222	229	236	243	250
72	140	147	154	162	169	177	184	191	199	206	213	221	228	235	242	250	258
73	144	151	159	166	174	182	189	197	204	212	219	227	235	242	250	257	265
74	148	155	163	171	179	186	194	202	210	218	225	233	241	249	256	264	272
75	152	160	168	176	184	192	200	208	216	224	232	240	248	256	264	272	279
76	156	164	172	180	189	197	205	213	221	230	238	246	254	263	271	279	287

APPENDIX B - BODY MASS INDEX TABLE 2

To use the table, find the appropriate height in the left-hand column labeled Height. Move across to a given weight (in pounds). The number at the top of the column is the BMI at that height and weight. Pounds have been rounded off.

BMI	36	37	38	39	40	41	42	43	44	45	46	47	48	49	50	51	52	53	54
Height (inches)								Body Weight (pounds)											
58	172	177	181	186	191	196	201	205	210	215	220	224	229	234	239	244	248	253	258
59	178	183	188	193	198	203	208	212	217	222	227	232	237	242	247	252	257	262	267
60	184	189	194	199	204	209	215	220	225	230	235	240	245	250	255	261	266	271	276
61	190	195	201	206	211	217	222	227	232	238	243	248	254	259	264	269	275	280	285
62	196	202	207	213	218	224	229	235	240	246	251	256	262	267	273	278	284	289	295
63	203	208	214	220	225	231	237	242	248	254	259	265	270	278	282	287	293	299	304
64	209	215	221	227	232	238	244	250	256	262	267	273	279	285	291	296	302	308	314
65	216	222	228	234	240	246	252	258	264	270	276	282	288	294	300	306	312	318	324
66	223	229	235	241	247	253	260	266	272	278	284	291	297	303	309	315	322	328	334
67	230	236	242	249	255	261	268	274	280	287	293	299	306	312	319	325	331	338	344
68	236	243	249	256	262	269	276	282	289	295	302	308	315	322	328	335	341	348	354
69	243	250	257	263	270	277	284	291	297	304	311	318	324	331	338	345	351	358	365
70	250	257	264	271	278	285	292	299	306	313	320	327	334	341	348	355	362	369	376
71	257	265	272	279	286	293	301	308	315	322	329	338	343	351	358	365	372	379	386
72	265	272	279	287	294	302	309	316	324	331	338	346	353	361	368	375	383	390	397
73	272	280	288	295	302	310	318	325	333	340	348	355	363	371	378	386	393	401	408
74	280	287	295	303	311	319	326	334	342	350	358	365	373	381	389	396	404	412	420
75	287	295	303	311	319	327	335	343	351	359	367	375	383	391	399	407	415	423	431
76	295	304	312	320	328	336	344	353	361	369	377	385	394	402	410	418	426	435	443

APPENDIX C - PERCENT OF OBESE U.S. ADULTS

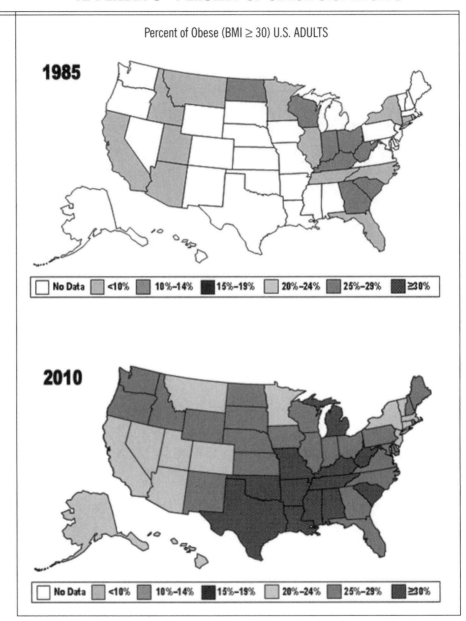

Percent of Obese (BMI ≥ 30) U.S. ADULTS

1985

No Data <10% 10%–14% 15%–19% 20%–24% 25%–29% ≧30%

2010

No Data <10% 10%–14% 15%–19% 20%–24% 25%–29% ≧30%

2010 STATE OBESITY RATES

State	%	State	%	State	%	State	%
Alabama	32.2	Illinois	28.2	Montana	23.0	Rhode Island	25.5
Alaska	24.5	Indiana	29.6	Nebraska	26.9	South Carolina	31.5
Arizona	24.3	Iowa	28.4	Nevada	22.4	South Dakota	27.3
Arkansas	30.1	Kansas	29.4	New Hampshire	25.0	Tennessee	30.8
California	24.0	Kentucky	31.3	New Jersey	23.8	Texas	31.0
Colorado	21.0	Louisiana	31.0	New Mexico	25.1	Utah	22.5
Connecticut	22.5	Maine	26.8	New York	23.9	Vermont	23.2
Delaware	28.0	Maryland	27.1	North Carolina	27.8	Virginia	26.0
District of Columbia	22.2	Massachusetts	23.0	North Dakota	27.2	Washington	25.5
Florida	26.6	Michigan	30.9	Ohio	29.2	West Virginia	32.5
Georgia	29.6	Minnesota	24.8	Oklahoma	30.4	Wisconsin	26.3
Hawaii	22.7	Mississippi	34.0	Oregon	26.8	Wyoming	25.1
Idaho	26.5	Missouri	30.5	Pennsylvania	28.6		

The data shown in these maps were collected through the CDC's **Behavioral Risk Factor Surveillance System (BRFSS)**, on the basis of self-reported weight and height. Each year, state health departments use standard procedures to collect data through a series of monthly telephone interviews with U.S. adults. Prevalence estimates generated for the maps may vary slightly from those generated for the states by the BRFSS as slightly different analytic methods are used.

IMAGE CREDITS

All photos ©Powell Lane Enterprises, LLC, taken by Mark Mabry.

Except

p. 31   ©Louis Ingram/ iStock
p. 23   ©Roger Harris/Science Photo Library/Getty Images
p. 23   ©De Agostini/Getty Images
p. 23   ©De Agostini/Getty Images
p. 23   ©Kari Lehr/Image Zoo/Getty Images
p. 200   Centers for Disease Control and Prevention